Done with Dieting

Done with Dieting

Lauren R. Shaw

iUniverse, Inc.
New York   Lincoln   Shanghai

Done with Dieting

Copyright © 2005 by Lauren Shaw

iUniverse books may be ordered through booksellers or by contacting:

iUniverse
2021 Pine Lake Road, Suite 100
Lincoln, NE 68512
www.iuniverse.com
1-800-Authors (1-800-288-4677)

This book is in no way intended to substitute for medical advice or consultation nor does it intend to diagnose or treat any illnesses or medical conditions. Consult with your physician before starting any exercise and nutrition plan. Beginning exercisers should start slow and gradually increase intensity.

ISBN: 0-595-33525-X (Pbk)
ISBN: 0-595-66960-3 (Cloth)

Printed in the United States of America

This book is for Rick, my best friend.

Contents

Introduction

My Story

Before I begin to outline what I feel is the best way to take total control of your health and your life, I would like to share my story with you. While writing this book, I was bombarded by an overwhelming amount of information about dieting and why it doesn't work. However, I didn't think it was necessary to include countless amounts of statistics for something we already know. *Dieting doesn't work.*

Not only is dieting completely ineffective at reshaping the body and losing unwanted body fat, but its physiological and psychological effects are severely detrimental. Starving the body of critical necessary nutrients has been proven to lead to health disorders such as osteoporosis, gastroenteritis, skin disorders, hair loss, and obesity.

Psychological consequences can potentially be worse. Anorexia, bulimia, binge eating, depression, and anxiety are psychological disorders that can plague the dieter for life. An individual struggling with any of these psychological disorders may never find peace with food. I am here to tell you that you can find peace and end the internal battle within yourself.

I began my fitness and weight loss endeavor at the early age of seventeen. I started working out with my Mom's exercise videos. I fell in love with the weights immediately and began reading fitness magazines and books whenever possible, trying to educate myself about weight training and nutrition.

Like many people, I also incorporated a vigorous cardiovascular/aerobics routine either before or after my workouts. On days where I didn't have time to do both, I always opted to do some sort of cardio exercise. After all, aerobic exercise was the best way to burn nagging body fat, and the more the better, at least that's what I thought. I wasn't alone though. Practically every source of literature and exercise video available reinforced the myth that aerobic activity was the best method for burning excess body fat.

Because I was never good at (or even enjoyed) doing anything that elevated my heart rate, this was a big challenge for me. Nonetheless, I pushed through all those cardio sessions. Running, jogging, stair climbing, and riding thousands of miles on a stationary bike—you name it, I did it. I would soon learn that the most important factor with weight loss involved proper eating and not excess aerobic activity.

Like most people, I did the low fat thing for quite some time. I believed that because something was labeled low fat, it meant endless quantities. I could justify eating a larger portion here and there because, after all, I must have burned hundreds of thousands of calories from my cardio, or at least it felt that way. Sadly, I was just spinning my wheels. Had I known that then, I would have ended all efforts for sure. Instead, I stuck to my routine like glue, believing I was on the right track.

My first real success with weight loss was in 1999. I entered the national *Body of Work* (now *Body for Life*) contest sponsored by the EAS supplement company. I was flipping through the pages of *Muscle & Fitness* and saw the contest advertised. I thought the contest challenge would be perfect for me because I needed a driving force to get me going.

I continued to do my usual routine, but focused on extra cardio and began taking fat burner pills and drinking meal replacement shakes regularly. I ate mostly low fat foods and counted every last calorie, protein, carbohydrate, and fat gram. For the most part, I was just having three meals per day, and either one to two meal replacement shakes per day as well. I snacked on fruit, vegetables, low fat crackers, and rice cakes. I also took a day off every week and ate pretty much whatever I wanted. (Note that this was before the *Body for Life* book was released, and there weren't any real guidelines to go by, except supplement recommendations.)

I ended up winning the *4-Week-Sprint* part of the contest and was thrilled to have made such amazing progress in a short amount of time. I finished the contest in pretty good shape, and for the most part stayed consistent with my regiment through the end of the year.

In January 2000, I moved away from home and began to settle back into my old ways. Pound by pound, I began to gain back the body fat that I had worked so hard to get rid of. Nonetheless, I enjoyed the break. I was no longer spending an hour to two hours working out and doing cardio. My priority was now on starting a business, which consumed most of my extra time. My food choices changed dramatically. I began to indulge in peanut butter cups when I was busy working at the computer—a few here, a few there, who was counting anyways? Before I knew it, I was *fifty pounds* heavier. Worst of all, I was depressed because my life was going nowhere, fast. My business ventures seemed hopeless, and I now had excess amounts of idle time.

I soon developed a terrible binge eating disorder and remedied myself with excessive amounts of food. I ate uncontrollably most days, and sometimes for no reason at all. I also began drinking more. What was once an occasional glass of wine, was now becoming two to three drinks per day, and continuing to escalate. I was out of control. The weight gain was just an everyday reminder of what I had been and what I was becoming. How could this happen after I had achieved so much? I wouldn't know the reason why for quite some time.

I continued this self destructive behavior until March of 2001. It was then that I decided to try again. The turning point for me was when my Mom was showing my transformation pictures from the 1999 contest to a family friend. I was shocked when I saw the pictures (which I had been avoiding) and knew that they were probably wondering what the heck happened to me! I knew then that I had to get serious. So I did. I was determined that this time around I would do even better than I did in 1999.

I worked hard, doing cardio first thing every morning for at least an hour. I did my weight training routine as well, usually lasting about forty-five minutes to an hour. I cut out practically anything and everything that had fat and tried to watch my portion sizes. I was doing at least one protein shake per day and also taking fat burner pills. I stuck with the usual three meals and two snacks per day, but my appetite was out of control.

When I ate my meals, I felt uncontrollably famished and my snacking increased as a result. I would usually snack on grapes, low fat crackers, string cheese, and maybe a little peanut butter with some vegetables. Nothing seemed to satisfy me though. I was going overboard on my day off, trying to make up for every craving that I had through the week.

After four weeks, I did my measurements. I was nowhere near my intended goals. There were minimal changes, at best, and after all that hard work I was very discouraged. How did I do it the first time around? Why wasn't it working for me now? I decided to increase aerobic activity to give my metabolism a boost. Eight weeks went by, and then twelve. I decided not to do measurements at my twelve-week mark and opted to try on clothes instead. Boy, was that a mistake! I had a pair of jeans that I loved and used to wear back in 1999. Surely they would fit, I mean, I wasn't expecting them to be loose, but at least be able to pull them up! To my disbelief, they didn't fit. They didn't even get past my thighs. Talk about discouraging! So I did what I knew would make me feel better...*ice cream*. The next day, I decided to get right back on track, like I had a thousand times before.

I continued to push through those hard times of exercising until exhaustion and fighting uncontrollable food cravings. My three months turned into six months. It was September 2001, when I decided, once again, to attempt to fit into my favorite jeans. I knew I had lost weight on the scale, and I was beginning to see the definition in my arms and legs again. I was both relieved and disappointed when I tried on the jeans again. This time they fit, but barely. They were so snug that I had to take them off almost immediately for fear of ripping a seam! But they fit! I was getting closer. But how much longer would it take?

Not much changed with my eating and working out over the next year. I lost a little more weight, and managed to wear those jeans again, but they never really looked quite as good as they used to. My life was changing though, and new opportunities arose.

I moved back home and decided to join a gym to further challenge myself. My weight collection at home was minimal and I had outgrown it. Being at the gym was a real treat for me because I had so much equipment at my disposal. I do have to say, I missed the privacy of working out at home, and felt pressured to look halfway decent when I was there. I continued to do my routine of cardio and weights. I was lifting heavier and began noticing more muscle development in my upper body. My lower body though, was another story. I just couldn't seem to shake those last fifteen pounds, no matter how much cardio I did.

I started to experiment with different protein powders, protein bars, and fat burner pills. Not only did my body fat continue to stay glued to my body, but now I was feeling light headed and noticing my heart rate randomly accelerating throughout the day (and I was taking the lowest recommended dose possible!) I was practically choking on protein shakes, and opted to eat the protein bars instead. I was in denial when I looked at the label on the back of a popular name brand protein bar to find that it had 13 grams of fat and 42 grams of carbohydrates. It had to be good for me though, it has *20 grams of protein.* So I religiously had one everyday. In hindsight, I would have been better off eating a *Snickers Bar!*

I met my fiancé, Rick in August of 2002. We began working out together consistently. I was getting stronger, and body fat was decreasing because of the added muscle mass I was putting on. Rick really taught me a lot about working out with weights. He taught me the importance of training intensity, which I already thought I knew everything about. After all, I had been working out for almost ten years before I met him. However, I really didn't understand intensity and the huge factor it has on increasing lean muscle mass. I was still doing my usual cardio routine before my workouts and pushing myself to my maximum capacity every time. I used to envy him because he could just walk into the gym without having to do a single cardio session. I pondered the thought of sparing that extra energy from cardio, and channeling it into a good weight training session. But I had resigned myself to doing cardio for the rest of my life, just like everyone else.

Soon after that, I began to notice that I was having trouble breathing and recovering after my cardio sessions. Within twenty to thirty minutes, my breathing would return to normal and I would be ok. Everyday the symptoms worsened, but I pushed through it. It came to the point were I would practically be gasping for air when I got off of the stair climber. The over-the-counter inhaler I was using to help with recovery was becoming ineffective. Even worse, was that my breathing began to change during the warm up phase of my cardio sessions. I was completely devastated. What was I going to do? I knew that I had exercise induced asthma, but I thought it could be controlled. I began using prescription asthma medication, but with no avail. My asthma symptoms progressively worsened. It dawned on me that I was going to have to quit cardio all together. After all, what's more important? Breathing or doing the Stair climber? Even so, I still couldn't help but wonder how I was ever going to burn fat without cardio.

It was during this time, a friend of mine that I worked with suggested that I do a local bodybuilding competition. I thought she was crazy. Me? A bodybuilder? I thought bodybuilders were supposed to be super lean and had muscles popping out everywhere. How would I ever enter a bodybuilding competition without doing tons of cardio? It *could* never happen. It *would* never happen.

Because I could no longer do cardio, due to the now permanent asthma I had developed, I had to focus on one thing in particular—eating. What I had been doing all along was wrong. Even though I was trying to follow some sort of eating regiment for weight loss, all I was doing was telling my body to hang on to every last ounce of fat. Pretty depressing, isn't it? And to make matters worse, the cardio that I was so adamant about doing was only hindering my weight loss as well. The extra muscle mass that I was trying to put on was just being metabolized to accommodate my body's energy demands.

And so the *real* transformation began. I eliminated all processed foods, ate lots of vegetables, began to eat every three hours, and drank lots of water. As a personal challenge to myself, and to this program, I decided to see how well the eating plan would work, by entering the bodybuilding competition. I'm sure everyone thought I was crazy or that I would eventually talk myself out of it, but I didn't. I refined my plan further and stuck to it like glue. I still had a day off from working out and eating clean, which I began to enjoy, rather than just smothering myself with junk food. I not only noticed immediate changes in my physical appearance, but my overall mental disposition greatly improved. I felt a new sense of confidence. It didn't just come from looking good (although that was a big part of it), it came from feeling good.

I started preparing for the May competition in February 2003. I stayed consistent, getting up at 4:30 a.m. to be at the gym by 5:15 a.m., five days per week. I took my day off every week up until the last four weeks. Before I knew it, May had arrived. But the best part was that I was *ready*. I did well in the competition, and it was definitely a wonderful challenge. I couldn't believe that I was actually on stage, in a *bikini* yet! I reveled in the fact that I looked this good, and not a single supplement or minute on the treadmill had *anything* to do with my transformation.

The funny thing about all of this is that it all happened for a *reason*. If someone would have told me ten years ago that I didn't need to be bothered with all that unnecessary cardio, and those expensive, ineffective supplements, and that I could do everything on my own by just eating good food, working out with weights, and staying consistent, I would have never believed them. So I had to learn this way. It was the *only* way.

The best thing about my journey was not just the change in my body, but the change in me. I have learned so much about myself, my strengths, and my weaknesses. I learned that I have control over every aspect of my life. I learned the unequivocal importance of accountability and personal responsibility. Yes, it took some time to get there, but it was worth every day. I came to terms with the bad habits that had plagued me. I no longer resort to food and alcohol to comfort me. I take pleasure in staying healthy, because I am a happier person that way. However, everyone has a unique learning curve in the quest for better health and fitness. It takes some people longer than others to realize and confront the underlying issues that are holding them back, and some never will. I can only share my experience with you.

"People begin to become successful the minute they decide to be."

—Harvey Mackey

Chapter 1

Done with Dieting!

Why Dieting Doesn't Work

*Americans spend more than $40 billion dollars a year on dieting
and diet-related products. That's roughly equivalent to the amount
the U.S. Federal Government spends on education each year.*
—*National Eating Disorders Association*

By saying that you are going on a diet inevitably means that you will eventually go off the diet. The entire concept of dieting is that you will be in a temporary state of restriction. But restriction of what? Fat...carbohydrates...calories? Most popular diets have some sort of plan that intends for you, the dieter, to return to some sort of normalcy of eating after the restriction phase. And what does *normal* eating imply? The return of those fats, carbohydrates, and extra calories that you had been painstakingly avoiding all that time? With a little luck and lots of willpower, it may work. But history has proven that this doesn't work.

The majority of dieters will eventually concede to their cravings and guiltily splurge on the foods they are not allowed to enjoy. Many justify and rationalize their temptations by committing to return to the diet and start over in some sort of introductory phase that puts them back at square one. What's worse is that most of these dieters will never reach the sought after normal-eating-phase, or *maintenance phase* of the diet. Instead, they will continue in this viscous cycle of deprivation and deviation and most likely drop out of the plan. Sounds dreadful, doesn't it? And if that's not enough to drive you to the edge of a sugar-induced feeding frenzy, then see what's in store next!

When you embark on your dieting journey, you probably are experiencing feelings of extreme hunger, sugar or carbohydrate cravings, and also periods of tiredness and exhaustion. You may find most of your thoughts are occupied with food, specifically pizza and ice cream! You remind yourself that it's a matter of *willpower* and continue to endure these hard times with your weight loss goal in sight. But what you don't know is that your body is fighting a losing battle that doesn't end with weight loss. Not only are you driving yourself insane with endless food cravings, but your body is now programming itself to slow down metabolically by trying to conserve all extra energy. This energy that I am referring to is fat—the very thing you are trying to rid yourself of.

So why does your metabolism slow down? Shouldn't it be burning more calories and body fat since you are restricting yourself? Less is more, right? *Wrong!* Your body at all times is in *survival or starvation mode*. This is a genetic predisposition that we all have. Most people tend to hold on to a certain amount of body fat for *survival* reasons, meaning your body is saving this extra energy, in the form of fat, for a rainy day. In case of famine, which is highly unlikely in this country, your body can then utilize its body fat for energy. This may seem archaic, but it was quite necessary at one time. As we evolved, however, this trait has seemingly stayed put. While your mind may have the greatest intentions coupled with willpower of steel, it cannot reverse this trait.

By restricting caloric intake, the body signals itself to slow things down because there is not enough energy, in the form of food, coming in. All metabolic processes slow down including body fat metabolism or *ketosis*—the body's method of using its own fat for energy. And, if you find yourself skipping meals in the quest to speed up your weight loss, you will have an even slower metabolic rate. At this point, you have primed your body for weight gain. But there is hope, as you will learn.

The Dieter's Cycle

Dieting forces your body into starvation mode. It responds by slowing down many of its normal functions to conserve energy. This means your natural metabolism actually slows down.

—*National Eating Disorders Association*

There are many consequences to going on and off diets, or *yo-yo dieting* as it is commonly referred to. Psychological effects are perhaps the worst. The mentality of starting a diet usually leads the dieter to have thoughts of deprivation that can be quite difficult to overcome. For example, the ever popular *low* or *no carbohydrate* plans emphasize the temporary or permanent restriction of essential carbohydrates. Many dieters attempt these types of plans with little or no success. This extreme restriction of carbohydrates is just too overwhelming, and many find themselves hopelessly binging out of control.

Other diets may emphasize overall caloric restriction. These dieters find themselves overwhelmed with hunger and inevitably overeat. The end result of both types of diets is *deviation*. Most often a deviation is not minor, unless you are one of the few people left in the world that can eat *just one* potato chip (not likely). If you're like me, it usually amounts to something like a quart of ice cream, cheeseburger, liter of soda, five cookies, and a handful of potato chips. In the end you are left with feelings of guilt, failure, and self loathing, not to mention empty cupboards. For many dieter's, the overwhelming feelings of failure combined with the mounting pressure to be thin, can lead to debilitating psychological eating disorders. Binge eating, anorexia nervosa, and bulimia nervosa, are common disorders that many people become plagued with. Most often it may take years of therapy and counseling for many people to overcome these disorders, all of which are rooted from dieting.

The physiological effects of dieting and yo-yo dieting are equally as harsh. Starvation mode leads to the storage of excess body fat. The body's metabolism has now slowed to an idle. Deviation leads to excess weight gain and an even *slower* metabolism. After all the hard work you put into staying on your diet, and even the weight you might have already lost, is now back and then some, for a rainy day, of course.

The last phase of the dieter's cycle results in either repeating the cycle and subsequently putting on even more weight with each attempt, or giving up completely. It's also important to note that 95% of all dieter's will regain their lost weight within one to five years.[1]

The Dieter's Cycle

Phase 1:
Starting a diet. Metabolism slows down
due to lower caloric intake and
decreased frequency of eating, referred
to as **starvation mode.**

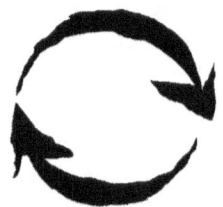

Phase 4:
Deciding to start over
again, go back to Phase
1 or give up completely.

Phase 2:
Feelings of deprivation and
excessive thoughts of food.

Phase 3:
Deviation, feelings of guilt and failure.
Gained weight back and possibly
excess weight from slow metabolism
and previous yo-yo dieting.

The bottom line is that it is unrealistic and unhealthy to try to deprive the body of the essential foods we need to properly function mentally and physically.

1. National Eating Disorders Association, *Statistics: Eating Disorders and their Precursors,* http://www.nationaleatingdisorders.org

Promises, Challenges & Rewards

Have you ever made a promise to a friend or family member and then broke that promise? It has to be one of the worst feelings in the world when you tell someone that you are going to do something and then don't. It is the ultimate feeling of failure and disappointment. How about when you make a promise to yourself and don't follow through? You probably don't feel nearly as bad when you change your mind and decide not to honor your own promise.

The truth is that whether you make a promise to yourself or someone else, it's no different. Over time, empty promises culminate into an overwhelming sense of self doubt and emptiness, knowing that you are unable to keep your word to the one person that matters the most—*you*. Start respecting your promises. If you say you are going to do something, *then do it*. If you want to change your life, *then do it*. If you want to change the way you look and feel, *then do it*. I'm not saying it's easy, by any means, but nothing worth having in this life is.

When you fulfill promises to yourself, you will find no better feeling in the world. Apply this utmost important principle to your life, and you will find a new realm of opportunities awaiting you.

Challenges are equally important as promises. Challenges are different, however. A promise you keep no matter what. A challenge is a goal, something to strive for. Challenges can, and should be met, but promises should always be fulfilled. Challenges, can outwardly seem good or bad, and should always be embraced. There is a distinct reason for each and every challenge you face, and you may never know that reason. Some challenges may present hardships, others present opportunities. Nonetheless, look at the obstacles in life as challenges. You may or may not succeed, but the experience learned along the way is the real gift. Use your challenges as stepping stones to your ultimate destination.

Challenges are nothing without rewards. Having a reward for a job well done is the key to your continued productivity and success. As children, we are taught that if we do something good, we will be rewarded. This reward can be tangible or intangible. It could be praise, it could be a toy, or it could be a cookie. The point is that we give children everyday challenges to prepare them for the challenges presented later in life. And to make them feel worthwhile, and to keep them working towards a goal, we reward them. Apply this same principle to your life. Set goals for yourself and work hard to attain them, and always, always, reward yourself. I will discuss the power of setting goals at the end of the chapter.

Find Out Why You Eat What You Eat

There are many different reasons for eating, and hunger is just one of them. Most often food is being used to fill some sort of void within us. Food gives us that temporary fix that we need to satisfy a deeper emotional craving. Start recognizing the differences between physical hunger and emotional hunger. Your body doesn't know the difference, so this will have to be determined in your mind. If you have already eaten lunch, for example, and you find yourself searching your cabinets for more, *take action*. If you are bored, recognize this and occupy yourself with other activities like reading, walking, yoga, gardening, playing with the kids or walking your dog. Call or visit a friend. Be proactive and you will find your cravings will pass.

Recognize that food is *not* the enemy. By truly realizing the importance of food as fuel for our bodies and not the source of your emotional emptiness can be a remarkable lesson. It is that type of *accountability* to yourself that you will need to instill to become successful. No one can do this for you. Confront the issues that are driving you to eat and face them head on. Don't make any more excuses or try to rationalize your reasons for eating. Make this your number one priority and you *will* be successful.

Setting the Example

Every day, thousands of people embark on diet and exercise routines only to find themselves back in the drive-through line and back on the couch. The pressure to eat sensibly and exercise is always in the back of our minds, but we can't seem to follow through. Most often, lack of preparation is to blame. We run off in the morning with barely enough time to get ready, let alone prepare the day's meals. I always hear the *not enough time* complaint, and I am amazed at the amount of time we spend on tedious things like going to the video store, getting nails done, and especially, watching television.

It is time to set the example. Many of you have children, spouses, family, and friends that could benefit *greatly* from you stepping up to the plate. Even if you're the only one who takes your food to work, or the only one of your friends that doesn't drink, you will be better off. Be the leader of the pack. It is *your* health, and no one else can change it for you. Take charge of your health and your life. You will be amazed at how quickly others will follow.

High Protein, Low Carb?

There are lots of good reasons for including a higher protein intake into your diet. But there is a fine line between increasing protein intake and *too much* protein. Protein is essentially composed of chains of amino acids. When protein is the primary food source, these amino acids can be converted to fuel. Ammonia (NH3) is the byproduct of the fuel production, which in high quantities, is toxic to the body. Both the liver and kidneys must do the task of disposing the wasted protein, which results in increased urination. This increase in body water loss amounts to weight loss in some individuals, but it is not permanent. Because excess protein has a diuretic effect, electrolytes and mineral balance in the body are disturbed. Calcium is unnecessarily removed from the body thereby depleting precious bone density. Over time, calcium deposits in the kidneys and may result in kidney stones.

Protein in smaller quantities, however, plays a vital role in many essential functions such as tissue repair and growth, transporting nutrients to the blood and cells, making antibodies, and lean muscle mass development. Protein is also necessary for a balanced diet and helps to curb appetite and carbohydrate cravings by stabilizing blood sugar levels. But in no means is it necessary to take in excess quantities over 100-120 grams per day for women and 150-200 grams per day for men. Eating excess protein that your body doesn't use, due to lack of demand, will ultimately be converted to fat storage.

Carbohydrates are equally important in a well balanced fitness and weight loss plan. Carbohydrates play a significant role in balancing the body's metabolism, blood sugar, and appetite. Carbs make us feel good mentally and give us ample physical energy. It has been my experience that clients who do not take in enough carbs are sluggish and tend to have poor workouts, not to mention slower weight loss. But the controversy over carbohydrates remains.

Carbohydrates, proteins, and fats, all have a unique ability to help the body gain or lose weight, and they are all equally important in the quest for fitness, weight loss, and weight maintenance. One without the others will create an imbalance and deficiency in the body and will not lead to permanent results. For example, a diet that is too low in carbohydrates may lead to temporary weight loss, but inevitably the body's need for carbohydrates is too great, resulting in deviation and excessive weight gain. The secret to weight loss and weight maintenance is to find a *balance*.

Carbohydrates come in many forms, from fruits and vegetables, to refined foods like bread, pasta, and sweets. Carbohydrates are classified in two different categories depending on their chemical structure and how easily they are digested and absorbed: *simple and complex carbohydrates.* Just as the name implies, simple carbohydrates are composed of one or two sugars, while complex carbohydrates are composed of three or more. Simple carbohydrates can be further broken down into types. Fruits, milk and milk products, and some vegetables are considered simple carbs. Table sugar, syrups, and sugar-saturated foods like candy and sweets are also simple carbs. Complex carbs are foods like starchy vegetables, whole grain breads, oatmeal, some cereals, and legumes.

Carbohydrates have many roles but most notably are critical fuel sources for the body and brain and are required for proper gastrointestinal functioning. Upon digestion, all carbohydrates are broken down into their simplest form— *glucose.* Glucose is then released into the bloodstream creating a rise in the body's blood sugar level. Carbohydrates not immediately utilized by the body as fuel will ultimately be stored in the form of glycogen, which is basically a string of glucose molecules that are linked together. There are two storage routes for carbohydrates, either the liver or the muscles.

Glycogen stored in the liver and muscles undergoes a process by which it converts back to glucose, the primary energy fuel for the body. When the storage sites exceed maximum capacity and the body's energy requirement is low, the excess glucose is ultimately stored as fat.

While carbohydrates are essential to a healthy diet, the *types* of carbohydrates should be monitored. Carbohydrates have a unique ability to raise the body's blood sugar or blood glucose level. The carbohydrates ability to raise the body's blood sugar, depending on the length of time in the digestive tract, has an associated number that is compared to a baseline number of glucose, the purest form of sugar. This comparison is called the *Glycemic Index.* Glycemic index has been made popular by many fad diets capitalizing on dramatic carb restriction or elimination for weight loss. Many of these plans suggest that carbs make us fat. While carbohydrate *type* should be monitored to some degree, they shouldn't be eliminated. It's not necessarily the carbs making you fat, but the type of carbs you are consuming and not to mention the *quantity.*

Glycemic index suggests that certain types of carbs are broken down differently, and depending on how quickly they are digested will determine the amount of increase in blood sugar. Without giving you the lengthy scientific version of this process, this is the basic sequence of events that happen whenever food is ingested. Upon eating a meal that includes carbohydrates, no matter what type, the body breaks the carbohydrate down to glucose. Depending on the glycemic index of that carb, blood sugar is elevated a certain amount. If this rise in blood sugar is fairly significant, the hormone *insulin* is released from the pancreas into the bloodstream. Insulin's main function is to lower blood sugar levels. However, insulin also has a role in fat storage. This is another archaic trait that the body has since retained. Insulin signals the body to store excess carbohydrate calories in the form of adipose or body fat, in case of future famine. Not only that, but Insulin also tells the body to retain fat, and use carbohydrates for energy. So basically, high glycemic carbs, in significant quantities, are most likely converted to fat, and your body will continue to hold onto this fat for a rainy day.

Refined foods and *white foods* such as white bread, pasta, white rice, and processed foods, tend to have the highest glycemic index compared to *whole foods* such as fruits, vegetables, whole grain rice, and oatmeal that tend to have a lower glycemic index. The body responds well to these lower glycemic carbs and achieves a metabolic balance. Not only does your appetite stabilize, but you benefit from the excellent energy source that only carbohydrates can provide. By reducing the amount of carbohydrates, especially high glycemic carbs, the body metabolizes fat for energy. This reduction amounts to 50 to 100 grams of dietary carbohydrate intake per day. However, there are exceptions. Cooking foods can increase the glycemic index and total calories, and also lower the nutritional value (e.g. boiled vs. fried or baked). Combination of foods also influences the total glycemic index of a meal. Consuming protein with a carbohydrate will help offset the carbohydrate/insulin response, providing a better balance in blood sugar levels.

While glycemic index is important, it's not everything. Other factors influence the body's ability to store fat besides glycemic index. Activity level, lean muscle mass ratio, daily caloric intake, natural insulin levels, fiber intake, and basal metabolic rate all have an effect. It is also important to note that everybody has a different response to carbohydrates, and the glycemic index is just a guideline. By restricting or omitting a food based solely on glycemic index will *not* result in weight loss. As mentioned before, carbohydrates have a very significant role in physical and mental performance, and also, weight loss.

Most diets and weight loss plans today are lacking one important factor—*balance*. Balance is achieved by consuming all of the very important food groups that contain the essential nutrients we need to function efficiently. Any nutrition plan claiming that it is necessary to restrict or omit any of the five basic food groups should be avoided.

Weight loss and weight maintenance *will* result from a proper balance rather than restriction of foods. Metabolic balance is achieved when dietary intake combines a balanced amount of protein, carbohydrates, and fat. Again, it is important to consider the type of carbohydrate consumed. For example, an ideal balanced food combination would be a six ounce lean chicken breast; ½ cup cooked long grain brown rice, and ½ cup fresh or steamed vegetables. It is important to consider the usage of long grain brown rice versus white rice. Both have virtually the same amount of calories and even carbohydrates. But the long grain brown rice has a glycemic index of 50 and the white rice 98. Simple variations like this make all the difference in how your body will respond. But the balance is important to note here. Chicken, a good source of lean protein, combined with long grain brown rice and vegetables, which are both lower glycemic carbs, stabilize the body's metabolism by keeping the blood sugar regulated and appetite satisfied.

A meal consisting of only protein will not keep the blood sugar at normal levels, but rather at lower levels, leaving you feeling hungry and fatigued. Appetite will not be satisfied and will be stimulated due to the lack of carbs. Overeating occurs, and the excess calories, protein or otherwise, are converted to fat storage. We will focus more in depth in Chapter 2 on the importance of quality and quantity of foods with respect to weight loss.

The Downfall of the Low Carb Craze

Within the past couple of years, the low carb phenomenon has reached profound heights of popularity. Similar to the low fat phenomenon, low carb has become a way of life for many people. Not only are people obsessed with low carb, but they are extremely misguided. Food manufactures jumped on the bandwagon almost immediately. You can go down any grocery store aisle and find products with labels that say *low carb, net carbs, and effective carbs*. What most people don't know, is that these low carb foods are not regulated. The FDA hasn't determined any guidelines for low carbohydrate foods. In fact, low carb labeling is illegal, according to the FDA. Recent research on low carb foods has found that there is little difference between a product claiming to be low carb and the real deal. What often happens is that a smaller portion size of the regular version is just used and labeled low carb. However, there is little enforcement at this time due to the lack of regulation.

So how is a food made to be low carb? Manufactures claim that the amount of dietary fiber that is included in a food is said to be non-effective in raising the body's blood glucose level. Basically, the amount in grams that is said to be dietary fiber is then subtracted out of the total carbohydrate amount. The remainder number of carbohydrates in grams is then said to be the *effective carb* or *net carb* count. This is very similar to the previous low fat craze. The primary emphasis then, was to look at the number of grams of total fat and saturated fat a product had. What was taken out in fat, was added back in carbohydrates, offsetting any potential caloric reduction. This is the same concept with low carb foods. What is taken out in carbohydrates, is added back in fat, again offsetting any caloric reduction. What's worse, is that portion size increases as a result. People indulge in the fact that they are restricting carbs, and increase the amount they eat.

With the low carb craze came the advent of low carb sweets and candies. From name brand peanut butter cups to ice cream to hard candy, the selection is limitless. These low carb foods are often made with sugar substitutes otherwise known as sugar alcohols. Maltitol, sorbitol, and lactitol are the most common. These sugar alcohols are said to be ineffective in raising blood sugar levels in the body. However, sugar alcohols still contain calories. But perhaps the worst thing about low carb candies are the side effects they have. These sugar alcohols are not completely absorbed by the body and bind to water as they pass through. Extreme cramping, diarrhea, bloating, and gas are most notable, and it only takes a small serving to experience this immense discomfort. It should come as no surprise that lactitol, the primary ingredient in harsh laxatives, is the same ingredient used in most of these products! Still, people indulge in these laxative treats believing that they are unaffected by the carbs in these products. I have even been told by *low carbers* that there is an acclimation phase to the candies, and that the more you eat, your body will eventually get used to them! Thanks, but no thanks.

The bottom line is that whether a food is labeled low carb or low fat, they all have **calories**. Sugar alcohols and fiber also count—*regardless*. There is no getting around that processed foods will always be processed foods, regardless of carbohydrate or fat restriction. The reality is that in order to be successful in losing excess body fat, processed food consumption will have to be restricted. There is not, and never will be, a quick fix.

Why Fats are Fattening

Part of what makes this plan so successful at reducing body fat, is that the amount of dietary fat consumed, is kept to a minimum. I am not suggesting that you eliminate or omit fats from your diet at all. You will ingest plenty of fat just by eating lean cuts of meat, poultry, fish, and eggs. Occasional use of olive oil for cooking or salad dressing is just fine. This is an adequate amount necessary for bodily functions.

Fat has many important roles besides storage. It is a wonderful energy source, supplying 9 calories of energy per gram. That's over double the amount of both carbohydrate and protein, both supplying 4 calories per gram. You can easily see how an excess amount of fat calories can quickly add up and result in stored body fat. By limiting the amount of fat you ingest, you will signal your body to burn its own body fat as a preferred energy source, which is a wonderful thing. However, I must stress that this *only* works when consuming frequent, quality meals. If you overeat on carbs, protein, or fat, chances are likely that the body will save the fat and metabolize the carbohydrate and then protein. So, consistency is especially important here.

Not only is fat a great source of harnessed energy, but it is imperative for almost all bodily functions. Hormone production is just one of the major functions. If the amount of dietary fat is too low, hormone production will be taxed. Fat is also critical for digestive processes.

There are good and bad types of fat classified as saturated and unsaturated. Saturated fats are by far the worst. A fat or fatty acid is termed saturated because it carries the maximum number of hydrogen atoms. These types of fats are found in most animal products, dairy products, processed and fried foods. Consuming more saturated fats means higher cholesterol and increased susceptibility for disease.

Unsaturated fats are broken down into two types, monounsaturated and polyunsaturated, depending on the amount of saturation. However, the process of *hydrogenation*, whereby an unsaturated fat is converted to a saturated fat, is possibly the most detrimental. Not only is the fat made to be more saturated, but the shape of the structure changes, converting a *cis-fat* to *trans-fat* or fatty acid. Cis-fatty acids, or essential fatty acids, are found in naturally occurring foods and have hydrogen atoms placed on the same side whereas trans-fat has hydrogen atoms placed on both sides from the process of hydrogenation. Trans-fat is the worst type of fat and should be avoided. The best way to tell if there is a greater amount of trans-fat in a food is to look at the label. If hydrogenated fat is listed first on the label, then the amount of trans-fat in that food is higher.

Alcohol—Empty Calories and Slow Weight Loss

Not only is alcohol completely useless nutritionally, but it will also hinder your weight loss efforts. This is largely due in part to the *empty calories* that it contains. Alcohol provides 7 calories per gram, almost as much as fat. But these calories have absolutely no nutritive value, so they will most likely be stored. Not only that, but alcohol is also considered a depressant. A depressant basically signals the body to slow processes down (including the metabolism), the exact opposite of what we are intending to do. As you adapt to frequent, healthier eating, your body will become much more sensitive to alcohol. You will find yourself extremely tired and sluggish, making for poor workouts and decreased mental acuity.

There are *no benefits* to alcohol consumption. As far as alcohol's effect on lowering cholesterol levels and increasing HDL (good cholesterol) amounts, even physicians will tell you to take up an exercise plan instead. Alcohol is not a good alternative. It wreaks havoc on the body and mind. So it's a *no win* situation. My advice to you is to learn to live without it.

Calcium's Role in Weight Loss

Contrary to popular belief, dairy products will not make you fat. As I mentioned before, excess calories, carb, protein, fat, or otherwise, will make you fat. Many diet plans today suggest that by omitting all dairy products, weight loss is eminent. This is not the case. Calcium, found in almost all dairy products, plays a significant role in fat metabolism. Instead of eliminating dairy, choose low fat, reduced calorie varieties of cottage cheese, yogurt, and milk. Lactose intolerant individuals should use *Lactaid* to allow for consumption of dairy products. You can also get calcium from lots of other sources like dark green, leafy vegetables such as spinach, kale, collard greens, and even broccoli. Salmon also has a higher amount of calcium. It is preferred by the body that you consume calcium through foods rather than taking a calcium supplement. However, if your body just doesn't tolerate dairy products, calcium supplementation is recommended.

Recent research suggests that there is a link between fat metabolism and higher calcium intake. When calcium intake is higher, this suppresses the fat storage hormones, allowing fat to be released from the cells and be readily available for energy production. However, this is only the case when consuming lower calories and lower fat. Dietary calcium seems to be much more effective in reducing fat storage than calcium supplements. Not only is calcium significant for fat burning, but it is also necessary for bone density and muscle contractions. Proper dietary calcium intake coupled with resistance training is by far the best way to increase bone density and strength.

Why Supplements Don't Work

Dietary supplements, protein powders and other formulas are promoted as food substitutes for losing weight, as health aids and for a variety of other reasons. People are often confused or misled by the many health claims related to these products. Often just one research study or several poorly designed studies are used to support these claims.

—*American Heart Association*

We've all seen the advertisements on television and in magazines marketing an amazing pill or powder that reports remarkable claims with regards to weight loss and muscle gain. The spokes model's perfectly chiseled abs must have resulted from the product, right? *Wrong.* Supplement companies make millions of dollars each year from desperate people who struggle to look like the models who represent them. Even the models themselves will tell you that hard work, exercise, and proper nutrition are the key elements in weight loss and fitness. Don't forget, they are *paid* to endorse the company's products. What makes this industry successful is simply good *marketing*.

My theory on supplementation is simple: *Its all garbage...Chemically engineered garbage*. You don't need it. Whether it's a fat burning pill, *healthy* candy bars, chalky protein powders, amino acids, or meal replacement shakes, you'd be much better off without them. And if there was truly a pill or powder that was engineered to make you lose weight and firm up with muscle, wouldn't everyone know about it by now? Trust me—they wouldn't have to advertise it anywhere!

The other problem with supplements is that none of them are regulated! There is no governing agency that reviews the product's claims, let alone ingredients, and determines if the claims are factual. On top of that, most supplements have scores of propaganda that accompany their claims. The doctors, researchers, celebrities, and athletes that represent them are all on the payroll. Convincing testimonies accompanied with unbelievable pictures make it almost seem crazy to not get on board. The American Dietetic Association (ADA) takes the same position: "As the research and interest in sport nutrition has increased, so has the sale of ergogenic aids, supplements, herbal preparations, and diet aids, all aimed at improving sports performance. The manufacturers of these products frequently make unsubstantiated claims to entice the athlete to use their products."[2]

The Dietary Supplement Health and Education Act of 1994 allow supplement manufacturers to use claims in conjunction with their products, regardless of whether or not the claim is factual. They are permitted to use any claim as long as it doesn't include or claim to "diagnose, mitigate, treat, cure, or prevent"[3] a specific disease. The other requirement is that the label includes all ingredients and active ingredients. Other than that, it is perfectly legal to claim or report anything about the product, whether it's true or not.

Bottom line, save your money! Weight loss and muscle building are solely produced from the combination of consistent resistance training and proper eating. Remember that the *cleaner* you eat, the *cleaner* you will look. Raw foods and vegetables will greatly enhance your overall appearance, including skin, hair,

2.   American Dietetic Association (ADA), "Position of the American Dietetic Association, Dieticians of Canada, and the American College of Sports Medicine: Nutrition and Athletic Performance," *Journal of the American Dietetic Association* 100 (2000): 1543.

3.   U. S. Food and Drug Administration, Center for Food Safety and Applied Nutrition, *Dietary Supplement Health and Education Act of 1994*, 1 December 1995, *http://www.vm.cfsan.fda.gov/~dms/dietsupp.html* (1 December 1995).

and nails. You will also be benefiting from all of the vitamins, minerals, and nutrients that are best provided by food. If you are eating properly, there should be no reason at all to include any sort of supplementation into your routine.

Natural vs. Unnatural Nutrients

Since the beginning of time we have relied on organic foods to survive. As we evolved, foods became domesticated and refined to suit our discriminating palates. We began engineering fatty and sugar-laden foods. We adapted to things like potato chips, fried chicken, hot dogs, and doughnuts and cringed at the thought of eating anything green or a piece of meat that wasn't battered and fried. Not only has the variety and quantity of food we eat dramatically increased, but our waistlines have as well. These refined foods are completely stripped of all vital nutrients, fiber, and enzymes necessary for essential health and immunity to diseases.

So how does the body know what is natural and unnatural? This determination takes place in the intestines through the process of digestion. Digestion is a multifaceted process that actually begins before food is ingested. When hunger signals from the brain stimulate the stomach to produce *hunger pangs,* the body is beginning the process of digestion by secreting special enzymes and HCL (hydrochloric acid) in the stomach to prepare for digestion. While you are chewing food, enzymes contained in the food are released. The quality of the food determines how many enzymes will contribute to the digestive process. The more naturally occurring enzymes a food has means better nutritive absorption and digestion, resulting in higher metabolic performance.

After the food has entered the stomach, HCL and enzymes further break food down. It is in the small intestine where protein and nutrient absorption is prominent. There is no conclusive or unbiased evidence that protein absorption from chemically engineered supplements is effective. In fact, it is proven that supplement digestion is rapid, thereby decreasing absorption. Only quality dietary protein with naturally occurring enzymes has proven to be slowly digested and absorbed.

It is important to note here that many factors can hinder the enzyme digestive process. Overly cooking foods destroys the enzymes that food has. Whenever possible, eat raw vegetables, or steam them instead of cooking. Raw foods contain enzymes essential for slow, nutritive digestion and absorption. The body doesn't have to contribute much, if at all to break these foods down. In fact, *metabolism will increase* just by consuming raw foods! This increase can be attributed to the entire digestive process of raw foods. The work that it takes the body to chew and digest nutrient rich foods stimulates the metabolism to work harder.

When foods are highly processed or chemically engineered, the body has to overly contribute to the processing of these foods by producing its own enzymes to break down these substances. This puts stress on the metabolism to take a time out so that the body can manufacture the necessary enzymes to break these mystery substances down. Overall, digestion is rapid, thereby not allowing sufficient absorption of any nutrients. Furthermore, the more the body has to manufacture enzymes to break down processed foods and unnatural supplements, the slower the overall resting metabolic rate.

There are various ways of determining a protein's quality and absorption rate. Biological value (BV) is the most recognized. Biological value measures the amount and proportion of essential amino acids, the building blocks of protein, which are contained in a protein. Of the twenty amino acids, nine are considered essential because they cannot be synthesized by our bodies. A protein must have all nine essential amino acids to be considered a complete protein. Animal products such as meat, fish, dairy products, and egg whites are considered complete proteins. Partially complete proteins are from plant sources such as grains, legumes, nuts, and seeds. These types of proteins need to be combined with complete proteins to provide proper amounts of essential amino acids.

Incomplete proteins consist of fruits and vegetables. These types of foods have very insufficient amounts of essential amino acids. The BV scale ranks whole eggs as the top source of protein with 93.7 out of 100, the highest ranking possible. Here are some other foods ranked by biological value:

Whole egg	93.7
Milk	84.5
Fish	76.0
Beef	74.3
Soybeans	72.8
Rice, polished	64.0
Wheat, whole	64.0
Corn	60.0
Beans, dry	58.0

Food and Agriculture Organization of the United Nations. The Amino Acid Content of Foods and Biological Data on Proteins. Nutritional Study #24. Rome (1970). UNIPUB, Inc., 4611-F Assembly Drive, Lanham, MD 20706

There has been no conclusive evidence that taking any protein supplements or amino acids enhances protein absorption. In fact, it is quite the opposite. As mentioned before, digestion of artificial supplements is rapid and converted to waste, or worse, body fat.

The Power of Antioxidants

Antioxidants play a key role in every bodily function. Antioxidants protect compounds in the body from free radical damage. Free radicals are essentially damaged oxygen molecules that attach to compounds in the body, like fats, and initiate chain reactions that create damage to healthy cells. Antioxidants can inhibit cancer, heart disease, slow down the aging process, increase immune function, and prevent infection, all of which are brought on by excessive free radicals. When you are eating clean, whole foods, your body will have ultimate access to these important compounds.

Antioxidants are found in the nutrients vitamin C, beta carotene, and vitamin E, and also minerals such as selenium and sulfur. Foods that are rich in beta carotene are apricots, broccoli, pumpkin, cantaloupes, spinach and sweet potatoes. The antioxidant lycopene, found most abundantly in tomatoes, has also been shown to have powerful antioxidant properties that lower the risk of heart disease and some forms of cancer. Oranges and other citrus fruits have been shown to strengthen the immune system and inhibit tumor growth. Citrus fruits also decrease the risk of stroke. Blueberries and grapes also have antioxidant properties that have been shown to lower cholesterol just as effectively as cholesterol-lowering drugs.

According to the American Heart Association, antioxidant supplementation is unnecessary, as you can get all the benefits from your daily intake of foods. The AHA promotes a diet rich in fruits, vegetables, whole grains, lean meats, poultry, and fish to reap the benefits of antioxidants. The key to making sure that you are getting adequate amounts of antioxidants from your foods is to eat fresh fruits and vegetables rather than canned, frozen, or cooked. The process of cooking, packing, canning, and drying all seem to have an effect on the integrity of the antioxidants.

Making a Lifestyle Change

"Go confidently in the direction of your dreams. Live the life you have imagined."

—Henry David Thoreau

Many people believe that weight loss is simply a matter of *discipline*. You may have the best of intentions, but find that self-defeating behaviors get the best of you. It is **not** a matter of *willpower* though. This is a *choice* that you make for yourself—for your life.

Your decision to become a healthier, fitter individual has nothing to do with willpower or discipline. Instead, think of your weight loss as a journey and a lifestyle change—*a change for the better.* It is time to rethink the way you perceive health, food, and exercise. It doesn't have to be a battle anymore. Embrace it. Accept that you will permanently adopt these new behaviors and never look back. There will be no return to your old ways of thinking.

Change can be a scary thing, even if it's a change for the good. This pertains to every aspect of your life. You will find that your likes and dislikes will change. Not only will you be looking and feeling dramatically better, but you will find that you have better mental acuity and focus. You will become emotionally balanced and stress will not have its usual effect on you. You will find yourself gravitating toward positive and likeminded individuals. Your entire disposition will change. This will take work on your part. After all, nothing worth having in this life comes easy, and this is no exception.

Setting Goals

"Obstacles are those frightful things you see when you take your eyes off your goal."
—Henry Ford

Goals are absolutely necessary to achieve results—*awesome results.* Goals are fuel for the fire. Goals make us work harder. Goals are what keep us driven. It is critical that you set two types of goals—*short and long term.* Short term goals are practical and realistic. This can be as simple as losing 20 pounds in 3 months or bench pressing 10 more pounds in one month. Other goals may be more health related such as lowering cholesterol by 30 points or decreasing blood pressure. The point is that there needs to be a fairly realistic ideal set with a means to achieve it. Have a reward for achieving your short term goal and do not accept it until you reach it.

Short term goals are your everyday plan of action. Stick to them and you will surprise yourself at how quickly you reach them.

Example of a realistic short term goal and *plan of action (POA)*:

What, Why, How, & How Will I?

What?

To lose 30 pounds in 90 days.

Why?

1. To feel better about myself.
2. To look better in clothes.
3. To be a better role model for my family and friends.

How?

1. Weight training program 3-5 times per week.
2. I will begin eating properly by consuming more vegetables, lean protein, and moderate amounts of carbohydrates.
3. I will eliminate all junk food snacking and replace with fresh, crunchy vegetables.
4. I will eat 5 to 6 small, balanced meals per day.
5. Water intake will increase to 1 gallon.

How will I reward myself?

1. I will buy new clothes.
2. Buy a new bike, weights, or walking shoes **or,**
3. Save the money I would have spent on fast food and dining out into a luxury vacation fund.

You can even set smaller, weekly goals. These goals should be easier to attain and may include things like:

1. Increase walking speed to 4 miles per hour this week.
2. Plan dinners and lunches on Sunday for the rest of the week.
3. Wash and precut vegetables for the week.
4. Decrease rest time by 30 seconds in between sets for all weight training sessions this week.

Not only will you add momentum to your progress but you will also become much more productive and efficient with your time. Revise your goals weekly and monthly as you accomplish them.

Long term goals are just as important as short term. This is the fun part. Before you begin, you will need to get into a relaxing, daydream-like state. You will need to *visualize*. The sky is the limit here. I want you to think of something that you would like to accomplish but believe it would never happen in a million years. It could be anything—looking fabulous in a bikini, taking a luxury

Mediterranean cruise, or starting a new business. This needs to be an ultimate goal. Cut out pictures of your vision, assemble a scrapbook, or keep a journal or diary of your thoughts and ideas. Find something you wish to strive for and visualize yourself doing it. Before you realize it, you will be there.

You will find that your body transformation is a journey. Not only will your physique change, but many things will change in your life as well. You will become much more productive. You will have a greater sense of self worth. You will be much more positive and find yourself associating with similar minded people. You will find that you will want to work towards greater things. You will have a newfound sense of freedom and finally realize that *anything* is possible. I can only tell you what I have experienced and several of my clients as well. This is truly a life changing experience. Don't just take my word for it—work towards it and it *will* happen.

Fact or Fiction?

Here are 10 common misconceptions about food and fitness…Enjoy!

Fact or Fiction?

1. All calories are created equal.

Answer: Fiction.

Calories are not created equally. There are good and bad calories. For example, fat calories, or the amount of calories coming from fat, are definitely something you want to watch out for. While the total number of carbs from a particular food or foods may be lower, the fat content may be higher. This is the case in many *low carb* foods. To make the item lower in carbohydrates, more fat is added. Try not to fall into this trap. Look at the overall picture. Is this food processed? Are the overall calories relatively low? Does it seem balanced? Remember, carbohydrates don't turn to fat. Only consuming more calories than you expend produces fat.

2. Eating a low carb diet will stimulate my body to burn excess stored carbs and fat resulting in weight loss.

Answer: Fiction.

Eating a low carb diet doesn't mean weight loss. If the total amount of overall calories consumed is higher than the amount of calories burned in a day, then weight loss will most likely not occur. Yes, it's true that the *types* of carbs that we eat vary significantly and can have an effect on weight loss. However, by restricting carbs, you will need to substitute other things, like protein and fat. These foods have calories too. If you're not stimulating your metabolism to speed up by eating clean and frequently, and incorporating resistance training, you will most likely store these calories, regardless of the type.

3. Eating small meals throughout the day speeds up the metabolism, offsetting the starvation effect.

Answer: Fact.

Eating small, balanced meals every 2 ½ to 3 hours will stimulate your body's resting metabolic rate to speed up. However, *consistency* is everything here! If you have one or two good days, and then one bad day, then this will not work. The body is genetically preprogrammed to store excess calories for a rainy day (starvation mode). It will revert back to this characteristic when you signal it to do so (i.e., skipping meals). So make this your number one priority and take food with you wherever you go!

4. Drinking a meal replacement shake or eating a high protein bar is the equivalent of eating a well balanced meal.

Answer: Fiction.

Nothing can replace the quality of a well balanced meal…*Nothing*. All supplements, whether meal replacement protein bars, powders, or pills, are chemically engineered. Supplements require additional help from the body in the form of enzymes to help break them down and be digested. This taxes the body's metabolic rate by slowing down to accommodate the production of enzymes. Digestion is rapid, and leaves you feeling empty and ready to eat sooner. Also, most of these supplements contain calories in the form of sweeteners, fillers, and preservatives. These calories count toward your daily intake, and chances are, you will add even more calories to replace the void you feel shortly after eating or drinking them. Take heed here. Go with the sensible, not to mention less expensive choice your body prefers—*food!*

5. I need a customized plan that is going to meet my body's exact needs.

Answer: Fiction.

The truth of the matter is that eating properly doesn't have to be customized. It would be extremely time consuming and tedious, to compute your body's exact caloric requirements. There are so many factors that determine this, and it can fluctuate day to day. I want you to start listening to your body and what it is telling you it needs. If you are hungry, you need to eat. If you are thirsty, you need to drink. Don't buy into the individualized, tailor-made programs out there. This is just another way for companies to market to consumers. Software engineers that create lengthy diet and nutrition computer programs have joined this marketing boom because they know people are confused and misled. Personal trainers that use this software plug in a bunch of erroneous numbers and a detailed report is generated. The client is then given an unrealistic diet plan that usually consists of very high and low calories days with strict rules.

These individualized programs promote the idea that the reason why dieters' previous attempts have failed was because their exact needs weren't met. This is *not* the reason. Fad dieting, and dieting in general, is the reason. The bottom line is that it doesn't have to be this complicated. Eating clean and frequently, and adding resistance training to your life will change *everything*, and it's that simple.

6. Dieting alone will not reshape the body.

Answer: Fact.

Dieting creates a reduction in the body's overall lean muscle mass and minimally reduces body fat. Remember, your body doesn't want to give up its stored fat, and would rather save it for leaner times. Instead, the body will metabolize muscle mass to meet energy demands. When you reduce your overall caloric intake and frequency of eating, the body slows down to conserve energy (in the form of fat). So your weight loss will usually come from a loss in lean muscle mass while retaining its body fat percentage, and possibly adding to it.

If you are eating frequently and have a reduction in caloric intake while increasing your activity level with resistance training, your body will respond by metabolizing stored body fat for energy and increasing resting metabolic rate. Not only will body fat percentage be reduced, but a shapelier, stronger physique will result—the best of both worlds!

7. Weight training will result in large bulky muscles in women.

Answer: Fiction.

This is probably one of the biggest myths of all. Contrary to popular belief, women will not build large, bulky muscles from weight training. In fact, it's quite the opposite. Not only will the ratio of body fat decrease as lean muscle mass increases, but your overall physique will slim down. You will notice this loss in inches by the way your clothes fit. You will also feel your muscles becoming much more firm and shapely. Strength will improve significantly, and you will find yourself with an increased amount of energy and endurance. The list goes on and on. The fact is, women need weights, and should train frequently and intensely.

As far as the stereotype masculine, muscle-bound woman goes, there is a very, very small percentage of the female population that has the ability to naturally build large muscles. This is due, to a small degree, to an elevated amount of the hormone testosterone that is present in these women. However; even that being the case, unnatural and illegal substances are almost always used in conjunction to create those dramatic results. So ladies, forget whatever you heard about weight training and *start lifting!*

8. Aerobic exercise is the best way to burn body fat.

Answer: Fiction.

Aerobic exercise is probably the least effective when it comes to burning body fat. You're probably both relieved and shocked to hear this, but it's true. Eating properly combined with frequent resistance training has the most significant impact on body fat reduction. Moderate to intense aerobic training has only a temporary calorie burning effect, and the type of energy utilized is directly related to the level of exertion and duration of time. Fat burning only occurs at low to moderate intensity. Good types of aerobic exercise at low to moderate intensity include power walking, bike riding, hiking, and weight training.

When you go over the moderate intensity level for longer than 20 to 30 minutes, the body has a higher energy demand. Instead of metabolizing fat for energy, the body resorts to the lean muscle mass to break down stored glycogen. As a result, lean muscle mass is metabolized and body fat is spared. What's worse is that because of the higher energy demands, appetite is also stimulated. You will find yourself fighting a losing battle while trying to control the body's overwhelming carbohydrate cravings. Most likely you will offset any previous caloric expenditure from aerobic exercise by eating excess amounts of calories to satisfy your appetite. My recommendation for a heart-healthy cardio plan is further outlined in Chapter 6.

9. I have a certain body type and I can't change it no matter what I do. I don't have good genetics.

Answer: Fiction.

We've all heard about the impact our genetic predisposition has on weight loss and muscle development. Is it really that much of a factor? *No.* The whole *body type* theory is also bogus. Once again, this is another attempt to market to the masses. If someone tells you that the reason you can't get rid of certain areas is because of your body type—that just makes you feel a lot better, right?

Yes, it is true that we carry body fat in certain areas more so than others, giving us the dreaded *apple* or *pear shape*. But body fat is just that—fat. Fat can be burned, and muscle will reshape the body, no matter what. So, if you've resigned yourself to having sloping shoulders, wide hips, or flabby abs, think again. Your entire body can change dramatically, if you work for it.

10. Weight training is the best way to improve bone density, lower cholesterol, blood pressure, and even combat depression!

Answer: Fact.

Not only is weight training the *only* way to reshape your physique, but it also has a myriad of endless health benefits. Bone mineral density dramatically improves because the bones have to adapt to the demands you place on your body from weight training. A recent study that looked at the effects of both mild aerobic activity and weight training and its correlation to bone density, found that neither aerobic fitness or mild physical activity had a significant effect on overall bone density. It was found that increased muscle strength was directly related to increased bone density.[4]

Total blood cholesterol also decreases because of the rise in HDL cholesterol (good cholesterol) that is produced by the body from an increase in fairly intense activity. It is important to note that exercise itself doesn't decrease cholesterol but rather stimulates the body to convert a portion of the cholesterol into HDL cholesterol. Consistency with activity along with proper eating will further reduce LDL cholesterol (bad cholesterol) and triglycerides, which are responsible for fatty deposits on artery walls.

Resting blood pressure also decreases with consistent physical activity. Depression can even be eliminated from weight training. Studies have shown that the hormone serotonin is secreted and elevated during and after a good workout. This leaves you feeling mentally balanced. Moreover, in an age where antidepressants are notoriously over prescribed, doctors should be pushing their patients to exercise more instead.

---

4. KJ Stewart, et al, "Fatness and activity as predictors of bone mineral density in older persons," *Journal of Internal Medicine* 252 (2002): 381-388.

Chapter 2

Why This Plan *Really* Works

Eating to Lose—Weight

If there is one thing you need to take away from this book, it's the paramount significance of eating frequently. I cannot overemphasize this. Eating frequently is a key element to successful weight loss and weight maintenance. Remember that the body is preprogrammed for starvation mode. For most people, fat storage is high and metabolic processes are slow due to infrequent eating (skipping meals), and overeating when they do eat. We want to change that, and the only way to do this is to *train* the body to think that it will always have food coming in.

Many nutrition plans will tell you to eat 4 to 5 meals per day. What they don't tell you is to eat every 2 ½ to 3 hours. The difference here is that you can easily eat 5 meals per day if you are an early riser, but you could easily have a gap of 4, or even 5 hours between meals. This inconsistency in frequency of eating can make all the difference in the world. The most important thing to remember when training your body to increase the speed of metabolism is to *stay consistent*. The body will naturally fall back into its preprogrammed patterns if there are extended gaps between meals that will cause you to feel extremely hungry, and be more likely to overeat. Consistency is a critical factor in creating an efficient, steadily burning metabolism.

It is also important to note that frequency of eating has a significant impact on muscle maintenance. If you go over the 3 hours without eating, blood sugar begins to drop and your body will begin to utilize the glycogen stores in the liver and muscles. However, these stores are very limited and are depleted fairly fast, mostly because the brain requires a significant amount of glucose for functioning. Once these stores are depleted, the body will begin breaking down protein from lean muscle mass to undergo a process by which protein is converted to glucose. Lean body mass is then slowly catabolized (the process of muscle metabolism) by the body to provide proper energy, offsetting the whole purpose of what you are trying to do.

So, no matter what, you will need to eat every 3 hours. The beauty of this is that you won't be relying on the clock to tell you when its time to eat. Your body will tell you. After you have eaten your first meal, your body should be *satisfied*, but not full. As you continue about your daily activities, your body will signal that its time to eat again. You will recognize this hunger signal and eat a nice balance of protein and carbs. The body is again satisfied, and you will continue this throughout the day. This could mean anywhere between 5 to 7 small meals, depending on how many hours you are awake during the day.

When your body is signaling you to eat with hunger, you need to respond. This is your body's way of saying that it is doing its job efficiently, but it needs *you* to supply it with constant fuel. Your body will stay on this schedule of eating and metabolism will greatly increase. You will have to be consistent no matter what! This will mean preparing foods ahead of time and packing them in a cooler. You will have no problems staying satisfied and on track as long as you are prepared. Make this your *number one* priority!

Eating Clean 6 Days per Week

Not only is it crucial that you eat every 3 hours, but you must stay consistent 6 days per week. This is critical. By eating *clean*, I mean eating good, quality whole foods and eliminating anything that is processed—anything. Every little thing adds up here. Even if you nibble on a couple of crackers or dip vegetables in peanut butter, this all contributes to the bottom line. Clean eating will dramatically affect weight loss and muscle tone, and also your overall appearance. Your hair, skin and nails will look fantastic, and you will radiate a much healthier appearance that only quality whole foods can provide. On a lighter note, you will be rewarded a day off for your hard work and consistency, which I will explain shortly.

Eating the Right Foods—Quality

Quality foods are vital to your success. Not only will you look better, but you will feel remarkably healthier when you consistently consume good foods. As explained previously, processed foods, including supplements like protein powders and meal replacements, tax the body's ability to efficiently process nutrients. Digestion is rapid and metabolism slows down. In addition, most processed foods are higher in calories and fat, further slowing the metabolic processes down. The key here is to allow the body to naturally absorb the required nutrients for muscle growth and repair, and metabolize its own body fat for extra energy.

Here are some examples of quality whole foods that you should begin substituting for processed foods:

Processed Foods	*Whole Foods or Better Quality Foods*
Snack crackers	Fresh crunchy vegetables
Protein powders	Hard boiled egg whites
Meal replacement shakes	Prepared balanced meal
Peanut butter	Light yogurt
Coffee creamer	Fat free milk or omit completely
Soda	*Splenda*-sweetened soda or flavored water
Rice cakes	Fresh fruit or slice of whole grain bread
White rice	Whole grain brown rice
Flour tortillas	Corn tortillas or whole grain tortillas
Cereal	Oatmeal—whole oat variety
Canned soup	Homemade soup
Pasta	*No Yolks* egg noodles or omit completely
Packaged lunchmeat	Fresh sliced chicken or turkey breast
Frozen dinners	Leftovers from a homemade dinner
Beef jerky	Fresh jerky made with food dehydrator
White bread	Whole grain bread

How do you tell if a food is quality? Unless it fresh produce, seafood, and meat, take a look at the back of the label. If there is more than one unusual looking ingredient or things that you just can't pronounce, chances are it is processed. There are some exceptions here. Some dairy products like cottage cheese and yogurt are acceptable and are also great sources of calcium. Try to stay away from fat free varieties of dairy products, which tend to be overly processed with lots of different fillers. Always choose the *lighter* versions instead.

Also, look for additives like MSG and preservatives found in canned or frozen products. Anything that needs to be preserved is no good, and should be avoided. Use some good judgment here and avoid convenience items. Remember, you are what you eat. The cleaner you eat, the cleaner you will look.

Eating Frequently—Quantity

As mentioned earlier, frequency of eating has a dramatic effect on weight loss and increased metabolic functioning. However, consistency cannot be overemphasized. You can't have three good days of eating properly and then have one or two bad days. Your body will respond to the frequent, small meals by increasing its overall metabolic rate. The number of meals you consume will depend on how early you get up and when you go to bed, usually 5 to 7 meals.

Every meal should be relatively small and balanced with a protein/carb combination. Some good examples are:

6:00 a.m.—Breakfast:
4 egg whites with 1 whole egg (scrambled), ½ cup cooked oatmeal (whole oat variety) sweetened with *Splenda*.

9:00 a.m.—Mid a.m. meal:
½ cup low fat cottage cheese mixed with 1 sliced nectarine sweetened with Splenda.

12:00 p.m.—Lunch:
6-8 ounce lean, grilled or baked chicken breast; 1 cup salad mix with extra fresh veggies like cucumbers, radishes, celery, etc., 2 tablespoons fresh balsamic vinaigrette dressing, ½ medium sweet potato baked with fat free butter spray and pumpkin pie spice (only 1 serving per day).

3:00 p.m.—Mid p.m. meal:
6 ounce light variety yogurt, 2 hard boiled egg whites with dash of salt and pepper, or albacore tuna salad prepared with fat free mayo served with crunchy vegetables.

6:00 p.m.—Dinner:
6-8 ounce lean, grilled, seasoned steak; 1 cup salad mix, 1 baked red potato, or ½ cup cooked whole grain rice (only 1 serving per day).

9:00 p.m.—Late evening meal:
2 or 3 hard boiled egg whites with ½ medium fresh sliced cucumber and salt and pepper, or 6 ounce light yogurt.

Contrary to popular belief, eating past 6 p.m. is good and necessary. Remember, you are programming your body to speed up and frequency of eating is critical. When you sleep for 8 hours or so, you go into a short term fasting state. Don't let this period exceed 8 to 10 hours. Your body won't turn your late evening meal into fat as previously believed, so make sure you get this meal in. Your body will still be burning calories, even while you are sleeping! A more detailed eating plan is outlined in Chapter 5.

No Carbohydrate, Fat, Protein, or Calorie Counting!

There is absolutely no need to monitor your calories, protein, fat, or carb intake with this plan. The focus should be on eating small, balanced meals 5 to 7 times per day. That's it. Why bother yourself with any other tedious details. Channel that busywork into creating new meal ideas, preparing your daily meals, and your training sessions.

You will notice that the recipes in this book don't have nutritional facts. It was intended that way. It's not necessary to compute every last gram of this and that. I want you to begin to choose clean, balanced foods, and consider portion sizes rather than trying to figure out how many grams of carbs or calories every ounce of food contains. Most often, people believe that if they can have so many calories or grams of something each day, then they can try to squeeze some junk food in and cut calories somewhere else. Save all that stuff for your day off.

However, I would like you to look at labels for your reference. This is a good way to determine if something is processed. If you see more than one suspicious looking ingredient, chances are its processed. Use the guide below to help you determine what is or is not processed. When in doubt, go with *fresh* fruits, vegetables, meats, and fish, versus conveniently prepared items.

Its processed if:	*Some exceptions:*
Its in a can	Canned vegetables, tuna, fruit (in fruit juice), canned tomatoes, tomato sauce, tomato paste, low sodium chicken and beef broth
Its in a bottle or jar	Nonfat mayo, nonfat salad dressings, most marinades (low fat or no fat versions), *all in limited quantities*
Its in a box other packaging	Oatmeal, cream of wheat, whole grain rice, *or Splenda*, spices
Its frozen	Frozen fruit or vegetables
Its precooked	Shrimp or other seafood, deli rotisserie chickens (skin removed, white meat only)
Its preserved	Some items like 95% fat free turkey bacon and deli sliced lunchmeat are good alternatives
Its microwavable	Healthy leftovers

Taking a Day Off and Why this Helps Your Weight Loss

A very exciting and also *essential* part of this plan is taking one day off a week to enjoy other foods. So, what qualifies as a *day off*? A free-for-all food party? No, sorry. Use some moderation here. The day off will only work if you don't go overboard. There are a few important rules to keep in mind regarding your day off.

1. Eat clean and consistent 6 days per week. Then take your day off on the 7th day.

2. Drink 1 gallon of water as usual.

3. Eat in moderation, but don't overdo it. **Enjoy this day, you worked hard!**

The day off is important for both psychological and physiological reasons. Psychologically, having a day off allows you the freedom to know that you can enjoy the foods that you love. Any plan that tells you to give up and abandon your favorite foods forever is just not realistic. Food is a wonderful thing, and to say that you can never have ice cream, pizza or enchiladas again, or until a certain phase of a program is crazy. Food is fun! Enjoy your day off and consider it your reward for a job well done. You will be more likely to stay consistent and less likely to deviate through the week because of the day off.

Not only does the day off keep you satisfied and on track, but it also helps keep your body's metabolism running steadily. Physiologically, your body will begin to adapt to clean and consistent eating. By taking your day off, you are essentially shocking the body and triggering it to burn a little faster. Your metabolism has been content burning your usual consumption of clean, healthful foods, and now there is extra fat and calories to deal with. So what does it do? It speeds up to accommodate for this increase in caloric intake. This *really* works! I must stress, however, this is only temporary. You must only take 1 day per week and no more. It will most certainly backfire on you if you push your luck.

Also, remember to consume your usual gallon of water as this will offset any fluid retention you may have from increased sodium intake and keep metabolic processes running smooth. The next day you will get right back on track, consuming clean foods and eating every 3 hours. Your body will be burning a little faster to recover from the day off, and the clean eating will be welcomed and refreshing.

It is this cycle, 6 days on, 1 day off that you should always follow. Try not to think in terms of a week, meaning that if you have your day off on Saturday, you can't have your next day off on the following Wednesday, just because it falls into the next week. Stay consistent, enjoy eating, whether it's your day off or not, and your body will respond with great results!

Why Your Body Would Rather Have Real Foods vs. Supplements

As I discussed earlier, the body's response to supplements is to digest them rapidly, which greatly decreases the chance that any nutrients will be absorbed. As a result, appetite increases because of rapid digestion. Metabolic functions slow down because of the body's requirement to contribute to the digestive process. In the end, you are left feeling hungry for more and working against what you are trying to do.

Raw foods have the opposite effect on metabolism and digestion. Not only does digestion slow down, leaving you feeling satisfied, but also the body doesn't have to work nearly as hard to digest these foods, and allows the natural enzymes found in the foods do the work. This allows the metabolism to focus on overall caloric expenditure instead.

Your body will naturally metabolize its own body fat for energy, and that's the purpose of this plan. Fat burning pills do absolutely nothing for you and are dangerous. Many contain herbs that have harmful side effects. Avoid these products in your search for the magic pill. There is none. Most importantly, remember that supplements are *not* regulated by any governing agency. There are no guidelines and none of these products have been tested by government agencies, so there isn't anyone responsible if they don't work or produce harmful results. Furthermore, there is no conclusive evidence that any of these products really work.

The Muscle Factor: Why the Weights Work!

Up to this point, we've talked about the importance of all natural nutrition and the role it plays in weight loss. While nutrition is a very significant factor, that alone will not give the dramatic effects that only muscle can give. So what does muscle have to do with weight loss? *Everything!*

If you've dieted in the past, you may have had some sort of weight reduction. Clothes may have fit a little better, and you may have lost some inches. Did your overall physique change? Probably not. Not only are you frustrated by all your hard work avoiding anything that tastes good, but also to look in the mirror and see only a smaller version of what you were. That's where muscle comes in. Muscle by comparison to fat is much more dense and compact, made up hundreds of thin, long fibers. Fat, on the other hand, expands and swells to allow fluid into its cells. Our bodies have a certain amount of both lean muscle mass and body fat that comprises a percentage of our bodyweight. An increase in lean muscle mass will ultimately result in a greater loss in *body fat weight* and inches, but also reshape your entire physique, giving you a leaner, sculpted body.

This lean muscle mass also plays a very important role in metabolic rate. The higher your lean muscle mass, the higher your resting metabolic rate. Basically, the more lean muscle mass you have on your body, the more fat and calories you will metabolize, because muscle requires energy in the form of calories to sustain itself. This means that you will burn calories and fat *constantly*, even while you're sleeping!

So as you can see, muscle has a profound effect on weight loss. Not only are you reshaping your physique, but you are essentially becoming a fat burning machine! Adding lean muscle to your body is the best way to increase metabolism.

So what about cardiovascular exercises like the stair climber or running? Isn't that also effective? *No.* Don't waste your time. Unless you're training to become an Olympic marathoner, high intensity cardio is absolutely unnecessary. In fact, it will work against you if you are trying to lose weight and put on lean muscle. Cardio sessions only have a temporary effect on calorie burning, and it really depends on the intensity and duration of your session. A recent study at Johns Hopkins University found that while aerobic exercise does burn calories, it is only temporary and the body's metabolism quickly returns to pre-exercise levels within 30 minutes. They concluded that resistance training leads to increased calorie burning for up to two hours following the workout.[5]

Your body needs to supply itself with energy during a cardio session, and for the most part, fat is an ideal source. However, if intensity is moderate to high, the body needs energy quicker and fat is not used. Since the availability of glucose from the liver and muscles is quite limited, the body breaks down muscle protein (catabolism) to make glucose to meet the energy demands instead. The body will continue to break down protein in the muscle fibers to provide quick energy to the body, and body fat is spared. Essentially, muscle gain will be much less because of this process.

In addition, moderate to intense cardio has an even greater effect on appetite. You've probably experienced this after a good jog or a spinning session at the gym. Immediately after your workout you may not feel hungry. A couple of hours later, your hunger is raging out of control. Why is that? Your body has depleted some carbohydrate stores and probably some muscle mass to fuel your cardio session. A slight elevation in metabolism occurs, usually during the session, but goes back to normal following your workout.

---

5. American Council on Exercise (ACE), *Lift to Lose Weight*,
   https://acefitness.org/fitfacts/fitbits_display.cfm?itemid=302

Because the body is depleted in nutrients and metabolism is elevated, appetite is stimulated. Most often, the body is craving carbohydrates to fill this void. Not only will you find it challenging to eat a small, balanced meal, but rather impossible. You will most likely overeat on good foods, which often leads to a breakdown on bad foods—lots of them!

Cardio, however, should have a place in every fitness and weight loss routine. The heart muscle is probably the most important muscle of all, and should have a workout also. An increase in cardiovascular activity has also been shown to decrease the risk of heart disease and cancer. The kind of cardio that I am suggesting is a good, brisk walk or bike ride three times a week. These sessions should be low intensity and about 30 minutes preferably. However, if your intensity is fairly low (you are not breaking a big sweat), then you can go up to one hour maximum, if desired.

Try to keep these activities fun and enjoyable without overdoing it. The main emphasis here is to keep the heart healthy and have a temporary increase in caloric expenditure without increasing appetite, not to see how fast or how far you can go, save that for the Olympics! The cardio plan is outlined in greater detail in Chapter 6.

Moreover, there is no conclusive proof that cardio elevates the metabolism throughout the day. In fact, it's quite the opposite. There is a temporary increase in metabolism during cardio exercise. However, it is extremely challenging to control your appetite when doing both resistance training and cardio. Energy expenditure is too high, and if you are following a lower calorie plan, your body will respond by catabolic breakdown of muscle tissue, regardless of your efforts. As mentioned before, appetite increases, and if you don't end up giving in to your cravings, you will almost certainly overeat by increasing portion sizes at your meals. Bottom line, you will consume too many calories and offset your previous caloric deficit from your grueling cardio session.

Resistance training has a profound effect on the body and is the only way to reshape your physique. More lean muscle mass promotes an increase in metabolism and overall fat and calorie burning. An increase in muscle mass creates a sculpted, leaner, and much stronger physique. Another added benefit is that over time, consistent resistance training refines your muscles. This means that no matter what age you start weight training your physique will continually develop and *mature*. Even with the same quality workouts, it is consistency that creates dramatically better results, year after year.

See Results in Just 4 Short Weeks!

This plan is designed so that you will start to see results almost immediately. During week one, expect to feel an overall sense of wellness following your workouts. The clean eating should be a welcomed change for your body, and you should feel this change almost immediately. Your mood and mental clarity will improve. You may feel a little tired immediately following your workouts, but this usually passes within a couple of hours. Your endurance will increase week by week thereby decreasing your post workout recovery time.

I highly recommend that you workout in the mornings, as this is the best time to find the energy for your workouts, and it also sets the pace for the rest of the day. You will be less likely to deviate from your eating plan knowing that you had a really good workout that morning. Week one is also a very important week for eating. Remember, consistency is the key to getting the metabolism up and running, and this stage is critical. It takes 21 days to develop a new habit. This is no different. Hold yourself accountable these next few weeks and make your eating and workouts a priority.

Week two generally consists of *feeling* changes in your body. Muscles are beginning to feel much more *firm*. Endurance is also improving. Expect to see the scale go down anywhere between 1½ to 2 pounds per week or more, depending on the amount of body fat weight you need to lose. Eating is becoming much easier as your body is beginning to expect the meals every 3 hours.

Week three consists of an increase in lean muscle mass changes. Exercise routines are becoming more intense and resting times are shorter. Eating should be simple and routine. The scale continues to drop and pants begin to fit a little better.

Week four—*wow that went by fast!* More noticeable changes are beginning to take place. You may notice your arms feel much more firm, and the waistline has become slightly smaller. Take a picture of yourself for reference and do measurements and body fat calculations, if possible. This is an important week, because from here on out, results really begin to compound and accelerate. Your mantra this week: Consistency! Consistency! Consistency! *Job well done.* Before you know it, you will be to your goal!

Don't hope for good results in 4 weeks—*expect them*! Think of your body keeping a scorecard at all times, *everything* adds up. This means that if you can get a couple extra repetitions in your workouts, or avoid all processed foods, even in small quantities, it makes a great difference! If you want to see the results fast, *stay consistent!* From this point on, results should become more and more noticeable. This will fuel the fire and increase your drive and determination knowing that your hard work is paying off!

Chapter 3

Getting Started

Make a Plan of Action and Take Charge!

"Nothing happens by itself…it all will come your way, once you understand that you have to make it come your way, by your own exertions."

—Ben Stein

It has been said that nothing worth having comes easy, and this is no exception. Deciding that its time to take control and change your life is a big decision, and one that you need to stay committed to. It will take hard work, sacrifice, and dedication, but what could possibly be more important?

As discussed earlier, you need to have a plan of action (POA) to be the most successful. Your plan of action needs to consist of both long and short term goals, your means by which you intend to attain them, and your reward for meeting those goals. You can be as detailed and elaborate as you would like, the main thing is to have them written down and in sight. Here are a few things to remember when creating your POA:

1. Have a clear, concise goal, and get right to the point. *(What?)*

Example:

I will lose 20 pounds in 3 months. (Short term goal)

I want to take a luxury Caribbean vacation next summer and wear a bikini on the beach! (Long term goal)

2. Give your reasons for doing this. *(Why?)*

Example:

I want to feel better about myself and be the best that I can be.

I am turning 50 this year.

3. Describe in detail how you will do this. *(How?)*

Example: I will begin weight training 3 times per week for 1 hour each session. I will take a power walk 3 times per week for 30 minutes. I will begin eating clean 6 days per week by cutting out all processed foods and incorporating whole foods instead. I will drink 1 gallon of water everyday.

4. Include any details and ideas that you have to keep you working toward your goal. *(How Will I?)*

Example:

I will begin a special interest class (i.e., foreign language, gardening, yoga, hiking, etc.) to occupy my extra spare time when I am usually bored.

I will take a power walk when I feel my willpower is low.

I will bring extra vegetables with me in the car or at work when I feel like snacking.

5. How will I reward myself for meeting my goals? *(How Will I?)*

Example:

I will go out to dinner to my favorite restaurant on my day off.

I will buy a new outfit every 3 months.

I will get a massage once a month.

I will put the money I saved on fast food and dining out every week into a savings account for a Caribbean vacation next year!

Just a little food for thought here, the average person can spend anywhere from $30 to $100 or more every week on fast food and dining out. In just one year, you could have saved **$1440 to $4800!** Pretty nice reward, isn't it?

The POA is critical to your success. Not only does it give you something to work towards, but it will keep you focused and on track for those days when you feel like giving up. Put some time into this and really think about what you want to do. Often times it's about *more* than just losing weight.

Get Excited About Your Upcoming Changes!

"Image creates desire. You will what you imagine."
—*J. G. Gallimore*

So your interest is peaked, and you're wondering where to begin. I spoke in the last chapter about the importance of visualization. You absolutely need to visualize. Whether it is an image of yourself strolling the beaches of Jamaica *(in a bikini)*, or wearing tank tops and shorts this summer, you need to have a vision of where you want to be. Even if you think it is impossible, visualize it. Be consistent and follow your dreams. You *will* get there.

You may find it necessary (and fun) to keep a journal or scrapbook detailing your vision. This is extremely helpful on the days that we all have where things are just, well, *blah*. Flipping through the pages of your journal will reignite your passions, and that's what it is for. So spend some time today on visualization.

Read Today and Start Tomorrow, Not Next Week!

Okay, so you've spent a little time visualizing your goals. Now its time to start! There is no better way than to just dive right in. I can speak firsthand about this. I spent way too much time planning for the day when I would get started on my weight loss program. I was always planning for the right time to start. Well I'm here to tell you that the right time *never* comes. The only one that is going to make any of your hopes and dreams come true is **you**—and although this may seem extremely cliché, it is very, very true. You will never realize those goals unless you do this, so make it happen, *time is of the essence!*

I am going to give you the necessary tools to help you get there. I want you to realize the importance of preparedness. As long as you stay prepared, you will always be ahead of the game and will see that there aren't any obstacles to hold you back. You have the power to do this, and it's as easy as taking 30 minutes out of your day to get prepared. After that, it's all downhill!

Shopping List—Grocery

I have compiled a grocery shopping list that will take the guesswork out of *what to buy*. Note here that you don't have to purchase all of these items, but rather the things that you will most likely enjoy. You will probably find yourself spending much more time in the fresh departments of the store, and not the snack aisle! I also advise that you don't shop for your *day off* foods. You will be less likely to go overboard on that day. Also note that this is the basic shopping list. See the recipes that follow and add the necessary items to your list.

Fresh Vegetables
Asparagus
Broccoli
Cauliflower
Carrots
Celery
Cucumbers
Mushrooms
Radishes
Spinach or green leaf lettuce
Red potatoes, sweet potatoes or yams
Zucchini

Fresh Fruit
Apples
Bananas
Berries: strawberries, blueberries, raspberries
Grapefruit
Grapes—all varieties
Melon—all varieties
Oranges
Peaches, plums, or nectarines
Pears

Meat Department
Fresh chicken breast (boneless, skinless)
Ground turkey breast
Turkey breast steaks
Lean beef and pork—excess fat removed
Fish
Jennie-O (or other variety) turkey bacon 95% fat free

Dairy Department
Cottage cheese—1% or fat free
Eggs
Egg whites—*All Whites (or other variety)* carton
Light yogurt—6 or 8 oz containers
I Can't Believe Its Not Butter spray

<u>Grocery</u>
Fat Free Balsamic Vinaigrette
McCormick's Grill Mates Teriyaki Marinade—great on chicken and turkey!
Canned vegetables such as green beans and spinach
Tuna or albacore tuna canned in water
Optional: *No Yolks* egg noodles for chicken soup
Optional: Whole grain brown rice or brown Basmati rice
Optional: Whole grain bread
4 cans low sodium chicken broth if making the chicken soup
1 jar low sodium chicken bouillon cubes for soup
Oatmeal—whole oats container or *Cream of Wheat*
Cooking spray—butter flavor or original
Diet Rite soda or *Crystal Light* drink mix

<u>Seasonings</u>
Splenda—sweetener
Pumpkin Pie Spice (great on sweet potatoes!)
Morton's Lite Salt (has less sodium than regular salt)

Shopping List—Training

Now that you have your grocery list, here are some items you will need for your
training routine. Note that this will depend on whether or not you will be working out at home or in the gym. You don't need to purchase top of the line on
everything, but make an investment in good, quality equipment.

Home & Gym:

Weight lifting gloves
You will want these to fit snuggly but not too tight. Your hands will have a ten-
dency to swell slightly when lifting weights. You should be able to grab a ½ inch
of material at the palm when your palm is open.

Exercise mat
Look for a mat that is between 1 to 2 inches thick. This is a good amount of
padding to eliminate unnecessary pressure on the spine and hips when on the
floor. Vinyl is also good because it's easy to clean and lasts a long time.

Ankle weights
These are fairly inexpensive and wonderful for adding more challenge to various floor exercises we will be doing. Start with a 5 pound pair (2 ½ pounds each).

Comfortable workout clothing
If you don't already have good workout clothing, you will need to get some. Find comfortable pieces that will allow for good movement. You don't want to have to be adjusting your clothes during your workout. Cotton works best for allowing adequate ventilation. Also get a comfortable pair of shoes with good arch support. Don't necessarily shop for name brands, but rather what feels best.

Home Workout List

Set of dumbbells—3, 5, 10, & 15 pounds
There are lots of varieties of dumbbells from classy chrome to neoprene padded. Go with what fits your budget. You might want to invest in a decent, sturdy dumbbell rack. This will make weight changes more smooth and take the emphasis off of your back.

Plate weights—(Two of each)—2 ½, 5, & 10 pound plates
These weights will be used in conjunction with the curl bar. These usually come silver or black plated.

Curl bar
This bar is used for lots of different exercises. It curves inwards in two different places for hand placement. The chrome variety will prevent chipping. You will also need the collars which secure the weights on both ends of the bar.

Weight bench
I recommend purchasing a bench that can be converted to both incline position as well as flat position. This will definitely increase the variety of exercises you can do. If that's not in your budget, a flat bench will be suitable. Look for a sturdy, well padded bench. A cheap, wobbly bench will be uncomfortable on your spine and limit your intensity and range of motion.

Wall mirror
Most people cringe at the thought of purchasing a mirror, but this is a critical item. You will need to see what you are doing as proper form is everything! Don't skimp here. Get a mirror that is warp-free and preferably shows your entire body from head to toe.

Optional Items:
Set of 8 & 12 pound dumbbells
Pair of 5 pound (each) ankle weights
Exercise ball
Exercise tubing with handles (medium to hard resistance)
15-20 pound straight bar (short) to be used with plate weights

Chapter 4

Preparation is Key

Why Preparation is Everything to Your Success

As you will learn, preparation is the key to staying ahead of the game. A little time out of your day will make all the difference in the world. I find it easiest to plan what I am going to be eating the day before. Take 30 minutes and plan your meals for the day and that's it! Of course, it may take a little longer to prepare certain meals. This way you're guaranteed to stay on track and be successful. You would have had to take the same amount of time to prepare macaroni and cheese or spaghetti. So either way, you have to make some time. Don't take this part lightly. It is imperative that you stay prepared.

One of the biggest complaints I hear is *I don't have the time.* You will have to *make* the time if it's important enough to you. Here are some helpful tips to save time and stay on track:

- Use a Crock Pot or slow cooker to make dinner. Some of the easiest and most delicious recipes can be made in a Crock Pot. When you get home, you'll have a hot, delicious meal and will eliminate the last minute impulse decision to get something *quick* to eat. The larger the Crock Pot, the better, as you will have plenty of leftovers for the next couple days.
- Pre wash and cut all of your vegetables on your day off and store in a large, airtight container in the fridge.
- Cook larger quantities of meat or poultry on the grill and refrigerate.
- You may also want to purchase a soft, collapsible cooler to take with you. This is a great way to keep food fresh on the go. Never leave home without having a game plan of where and when you will be eating. When in doubt, bring food with you!

Planning Your Week

Not only will planning become much more customary, but you will also find that you will be much more organized. Chapter 5 has a 2-week menu plan to give you lots of ideas and variety. I suggest that you plan your weekly meals prior to going to the grocery store. Whether you use the menu plans here or devise your own, get an idea of what you will need. Sounds simple, right? *It is!*

You should also have a workout plan for the week and stick to it. Chapter 6 will outline a home or gym fitness plan. Create a workout schedule and times that you will workout. Take these sessions seriously and consider them appointments. You wouldn't miss an appointment with a doctor or massage therapist, right? Well do the same here. Hold yourself *accountable.*

Keeping a Journal

Not only is a journal absolutely necessary to track your progress, but also keeps you accountable to something. Make your journal a priority everyday. Keep separate logs for food intake and workout sessions. Write everything down, even if you'd rather forget about it! This is a great way to keep you on track. I recommend keeping a food journal for 4 weeks and keeping a consistent workout journal. You may choose to keep either a notebook journal or make more elaborate charts to help keep track of your progress. The following pages demonstrate the simplicity of keeping a journal:

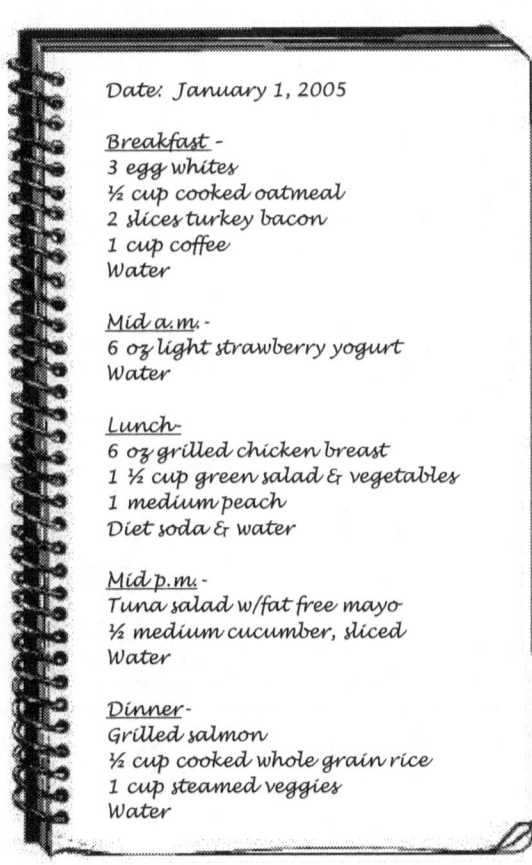

Date: January 1, 2005

Breakfast -
3 egg whites
½ cup cooked oatmeal
2 slices turkey bacon
1 cup coffee
Water

Mid a.m. -
6 oz light strawberry yogurt
Water

Lunch -
6 oz grilled chicken breast
1 ½ cup green salad & vegetables
1 medium peach
Diet soda & water

Mid p.m. -
Tuna salad w/fat free mayo
½ medium cucumber, sliced
Water

Dinner -
Grilled salmon
½ cup cooked whole grain rice
1 cup steamed veggies
Water

Date: January 1, 2005

Exercise	Set 1/ #lbs	Set 2/ #lbs	Set 3/ #lbs	Set 4/ #lbs
Dumbbell bicep curls	15 reps/ 12 lbs	15 reps/ 15 lbs	12 reps/ 10 lbs	10 reps/ 12 lbs
Preacher curls	10 reps/ 30 lbs	10 reps/ 40 lbs	10 reps/ 35 lbs	8 reps/ 35 lbs
Overhead triceps extension	12 reps/ 35 lbs	10 reps/ 45 lbs	10 reps/ 40 lbs	10 reps/ 30 lbs
Triceps pushdowns	15 reps/ 35 lbs	10 reps/ 45 lbs	12 reps/ 40 lbs	12 reps/ 35 lbs
Dips	15 reps	20 reps	15 reps	10 reps

Floor work:
Abs - 10 minutes
Inner/outer thighs - 10 minutes

Exercise	Set 1	# lbs	Set 2	# lbs	Set 3	# lbs	Set 4	# lbs
Dumbbell Bicep Curls	15 reps	12	15 reps	15	12 reps	12	10 reps	12
Preacher Curls	10 reps	30	10 reps	40	10 reps	35	8 reps	35
Overhead triceps extension	12 reps	35	10 reps	45	10 reps	40	10 reps	30
Triceps pushdown	15 reps	35	10 reps	45	12 reps	40	12 reps	35
Dips	15	-	20	-	15	-	10	-

Tips to Keep You on Track

Stay Full
You will be less likely to overeat at meals if you are always satisfied. Have extra veggies or fruit on hand to snack on throughout the day.

Be Prepared
Just as you wouldn't leave the house without your purse, briefcase, cell phone, or wallet, you shouldn't leave without food either.

Eat Frequently
Make sure you are eating 5+ meals per day. This is absolutely necessary to see results!

Eat Balanced
Always eat a balanced meal consisting of a protein and a carbohydrate. You will be more satisfied after every meal and are also providing sufficient fuel for muscle growth while stimulating the metabolism.

Drink Water
Here are some interesting facts about water:

75% of the U.S. population is chronically dehydrated.
37% of the U.S. population mistakes thirst for hunger.
80% of the body is water.

Not only does water make up a significant amount of the human body, but it is necessary for proper metabolic functioning. Dehydration can dramatically slow the body's metabolism down, which is critical to what you are trying to accomplish. The body will retain a certain amount of water, depending on your sodium intake, which causes excess bloating. If you are not hydrating sufficiently, the body will continue to retain water. Bottom line: The more water you drink, the less your body will hold on to. If your body knows that it will be getting water frequently, it will shed the excess.

Work up to a gallon of water per day. No, this is not too much! You need to drink half your body weight in ounces just to make up for daily water loss through bodily functions. This does not take into consideration *rehydration.* For optimal weight loss and metabolic functioning this amount is recommended.

Stay Creative!

If you are content with eating the same foods everyday, then you shouldn't have any problems with this. If you are the opposite, then put some extra time and energy (that you would otherwise use for something nonproductive) into being creative. Go to your bookstore or library and find low fat cookbooks that relate to this plan. There are tons of delicious, easy recipes at your disposal online also. You can even conjure up a few of your own! Creativity will keep you successful in the long run.

Chapter 5

The Food Plan

The Food Plan

If you aren't already aware of the huge importance nutrition plays in both weight loss and fitness, you should be by now. Results, whether with weight loss or fitness, are highly dependant on nutrition. So much so, that nutrition attributes to about **80%** of the results you see and feel. Yes, it's true, *you are what you eat!*

We've discussed in great detail the relevance of the types of foods that you need to eat and frequency of eating. The food plan on the following page is the exact plan that I give to my clients. Note that the sample menu plan is just that. There is also a more detailed 2-week menu plan at the end of the chapter along with a variety of delicious recipes suitable for this plan that can be exchanged for every meal. Experiment with different foods and have fun with it! Enjoy!

Let's Talk Nutrition...

You must:

- Consume 5-6 small meals per day, consisting of carbohydrates and protein.
- Eat every 2 ½ to 3 hours (stay full).
- Drink at least 1 gallon of water per day.
- Eliminate all *white* foods (no bread, bagels, pasta, white rice, cereals, and of course, sugar!)
- Snack on vegetables when hungry—vegetables are unlimited!
- Have a day off once per week!

Protein Selections

Tuna or albacore tuna
Chicken breast (skinless)
Fish
Lean beef or lean ground turkey (drain all excess fat when cooking!)
Turkey bacon—95% fat free
Eggs and egg whites
Cottage cheese—fat free or 1%

Carbohydrate or Starch Selections

Red potatoes, sweet potatoes or yams
Brown rice
Oatmeal or *Cream of Wheat*
Vegetables (broccoli, cauliflower, radishes, carrots, celery, spinach, asparagus)
Low sodium canned vegetables—except corn
Fruit (bananas, apples, peaches, pears, melon, strawberries, raspberries)
Whole grain bread—limit to 1 slice per day

Fats

Use cooking spray
Use *I Can't Believe Its Not Butter* spray on your vegetables and potatoes
You may use olive oil sparingly when cooking or in a salad dressing

Sample Menu Plan

Meal 1	Meal 4
½ cup egg whites	½ cup cottage cheese mixed with ½ cup fruit
3 slices turkey bacon	or
Slice of whole grain bread or ½ cup oatmeal	8 oz of low calorie or light yogurt

Meal 2
½ cup cottage cheese mixed with ½ cup fruit

Meal 3
Protein (roughly 6-8 oz, or size of palm)
½ sweet potato or ½ cup brown rice
½—1 cup vegetables

Meal 5
Protein (6-8 oz)
½ sweet potato or ½ cup brown rice
½—1 cup vegetables

Meal 6 (optional)
3 egg whites or ½ cup cooked chicken strips

Unlimited Foods

Below are a few unlimited items that you can have on this plan. Yes, unlimited means just that. You can have these foods any time and as much as you would like. Note that the chicken soup recipe is homemade, not canned or processed.

All green vegetables including:

Asparagus
Broccoli
Brussels sprouts
Cabbage
Celery
Cucumber
Green beans
Green onions
Green pepper
Lettuce—all varieties
Spinach
Sprouts—alfalfa & bean
Zucchini

Other vegetables:

Cauliflower
Mushrooms
Onions—red, yellow, & white

Radishes
Red pepper
Yellow pepper

Homemade Chicken Soup

3 lbs chicken breast, sliced into 1 inch pieces
2 cups carrots, sliced
2 cups celery, sliced
1 package sliced mushrooms
4 cans low sodium chicken broth
1 low sodium chicken bouillon cube
Salt and pepper to taste

Place all items in Crock pot, except mushrooms, and set to low for 6-8 hours. Add mushrooms ½ hour before serving.

Recipes for Success!

Breakfast

Oatmeal Pancake

½ cup dry oatmeal
3 egg whites or ¼ carton egg whites
¼ tsp vanilla extract
1 tbsp *Splenda* sweetener
Butter flavored cooking spray
½ cup berries

Add water to oatmeal and cook separately in microwave for about 2 minutes on high power. Remove from microwave and add egg whites, vanilla extract, and *Splenda* and mix well. Heat a nonstick skillet over medium high heat. Spray pan well with cooking spray. Take a large spoonful of oatmeal mixture and place in skillet. Cook approximately 2 to 3 minutes or until side is done. Flip and cook other side. Serve pancakes topped with berries and sprinkled *Splenda*, if desired.

Makes 1 serving

Omelet

4-5 egg whites or ¼ carton egg whites
1 whole egg
¼ cup diced green pepper
¼ cup diced onion
¼ cup diced mushrooms
1 small Roma tomato, diced
Dash of salt and pepper
Butter flavored cooking spray
1 tbsp green chile salsa

In a mixing bowl, combine egg whites and whole egg. Whisk egg mixture well. Add all remaining ingredients and mix well. Heat a nonstick skillet over medium high heat. Spray well with butter flavored cooking spray. Add egg mixture to skillet. Heat until the edges begin to bubble. Turn to medium. With a spatula, gently fold egg mixture toward center of skillet. When bottom of omelet is done, flip over with spatula. Garnish with green chile salsa, if desired.

Makes 1 serving

Fruit Salad

½ cup sliced fruit, any variety
1–6 oz container light vanilla yogurt or any other flavor
¼ tsp vanilla or almond extract
2 tbsp toasted almond pieces or other nuts (optional)

Combine yogurt and vanilla extract. Fold in fruit and top with almonds, if desired. Serve with ½ cup cooked oatmeal.

Makes 1 serving

Mid am

Fruit & Cottage Cheese Delight

½ cup 1% fat cottage cheese
½ cup fresh sliced fruit or berries
1 tbsp *Splenda* sweetener
¼ tsp vanilla extract

Combine cottage cheese, *Splenda*, and vanilla extract and mix well. Gently fold in fruit and serve.

Makes 1 serving

Smoothies

1–6 oz container light vanilla yogurt or other flavored variety
¼ carton egg whites
½ medium banana
½ tsp vanilla extract
2-3 ice cubes

In a blender, combine all ingredients. Blend well on high for 45 seconds. Serve chilled.

Makes 1 serving

Lunch

Albacore Tuna Salad

1–6 oz can solid white albacore tuna **or**
1–6 oz can white meat chicken or shredded chicken breast
2 tbsp fat free mayo or Miracle Whip
½ cup chopped celery
½ cup chopped green apple
2 tbsp chopped walnuts
1 slice whole grain bread
1 sliced small Roma tomato (optional)

Combine albacore and mayo and mix well until creamy. Mix in celery, apple, and walnuts and combine well. Cut bread in half, and served chilled tuna salad mixture on top. Garnish with a Roma tomato slice, if desired.

Makes 1 serving

Honey Mustard Chicken Sandwich

6-8 oz grilled or baked chicken breast
2 slices cooked turkey bacon, cut into halves
2 tablespoons honey mustard dressing (divided)
1 small Roma tomato, sliced
Green leaf lettuce
1 slice whole grain bread, toasted (optional)

Spread 1 tablespoon honey mustard dressing on top of bread. Place chicken breast over mustard and spread remaining tablespoon dressing over top of chicken breast. Garnish with turkey bacon, lettuce and tomato.

Makes 1 serving

Grilled Chicken Salad

6–8 oz grilled or baked chicken strips
1 cup mixed greens
¼ cup sliced mushrooms
¼ cup chopped carrots
¼ cup chopped celery
1 hardboiled egg, sliced
1 small Roma tomato, diced
2 slices cooked turkey bacon, broken into crumbles
2 tbsp fat free French dressing or balsamic vinaigrette dressing (recipe below)

In a large covered bowl, combine greens and all vegetables with dressing. Shake bowl to coat salad well. Remove cover and place sliced chicken strips, sliced egg, and turkey bacon over the top.

Makes 1 serving

Balsamic Vinaigrette Dressing

¼ cup balsamic vinegar
1 tbsp extra virgin olive oil
1 tsp finely ground mustard seed
Dash of salt and pepper

Combine all ingredients in salad dressing jar and shake vigorously before serving. Refrigerate any unused portion.

Makes 1-2 servings

Turkey Breast Burgers

1 package ground turkey breast (1 to 1.25 pounds)
1 tbsp minced onion
1 tsp garlic powder
1 small sliced Roma tomato (optional)
1 tbsp green chile salsa (optional)
Dash salt and pepper
Butter flavored cooking spray

In a covered bowl or container, combine all ingredients except tomato and green chile salsa. Mix thoroughly until all seasoning is combined. Spray nonstick skillet with cooking spray and heat over medium high heat. Shape turkey mixture into desired number of patties, approximately 6 ounces or size of the palm. Place patty in skillet and spray top of patty with butter spray to coat. Turn heat to medium, and cook for 5 to 7 minutes and turn over. Cook other side 5 to 7 minutes or until turkey is no longer pink in the center. Serve with sliced tomato and garnish with green chile salsa, if desired.

Makes 4 to 5 servings

Meatball Sandwiches

1 package ground turkey breast (1 to 1.25 pounds)
½ packet meatloaf seasoning or other desired seasoning
1 whole egg
½ cup dry oatmeal
1–8 oz can tomato sauce (divided)
1–4 oz can green chilies (optional)
1 tsp garlic powder
1 tsp finely ground cumin
1 tbsp dried parsley flakes
Butter flavored cooking spray
1 tbsp ketchup or mustard (optional)
1 slice whole grain bread
Parmesan cheese sprinkle (optional)

Preheat oven to 375°. In a large mixing bowl, combine all ingredients except only ½ can tomato sauce and mix thoroughly until all turkey and seasonings are blended. Spray nonstick baking sheet with butter cooking spray. Shape turkey into balls with hands and place on baking sheet. Top each meatball with a spoonful of remaining tomato sauce. Sprinkle with additional parsley flakes and garlic powder. Bake for 25 to 30 minutes, or until done. Sprinkle with parmesan cheese, if desired. Cool. Store in airtight container, and refrigerate.

Crock Pot or slow cooker method: Thoroughly spray inside of Crock Pot with cooking spray. Place meatballs in Crock Pot and top each meatball with a spoon of remaining tomato sauce. Cook on low 5 to 6 hours or high 3 to 4 hours. Sprinkle with parmesan cheese, if desired. Cool. Store in airtight container, and refrigerate. Serve meatballs with sliced bread and top with ketchup or mustard, if desired.

Note: Double recipe above for larger batch.

Makes 4 servings

Mid pm

Fruit Parfait

¼ cup sliced fruit, any variety
1–6 oz light vanilla yogurt or other flavor
1 tbsp low fat ricotta cheese
¼ tsp vanilla or almond extract
2 tbsp sliced almonds

Combine yogurt with ricotta cheese until smooth. Add vanilla extract. Mix well. Gently fold in sliced fruit. Top with sliced almonds.

Makes 1 serving

Homemade Jerky

1 package turkey breast steaks
½ cup Teriyaki marinade **or**
½ cup soy sauce
1 tablespoon Worcestershire sauce
1 tsp garlic powder
1 tsp finely ground cumin
Dash salt and pepper

Combine all ingredients in airtight container. Slice turkey breast steaks into 1 inch wide strips, lengthwise. Place turkey strips in soy sauce mixture or Teriyaki marinade. Shake well and refrigerate overnight. Place turkey strips evenly on food dehydrator trays. Follow dehydrator instructions for jerky cooking times. You may also use the jerky recipes that accompany the food dehydrator. Store jerky in Ziploc bags or an airtight container. You may double or triple the recipe for larger amounts.

Makes 2 to 3 servings

Italian Meatball Bites

1 package ground turkey breast (1 to 1.25 pounds)
½ packet zesty spaghetti sauce seasoning
2 tsp oregano leaves
2 tsp parsley flakes
1 tsp garlic powder **or**
1 tbsp Italian seasoning
1–8 oz can tomato sauce (divided)
(Try the basil, oregano & garlic flavored sauce)

¼ cup dry oatmeal
Parmesan cheese sprinkle (optional)
Butter flavored cooking spray

Preheat oven to 375°. Combine all ingredients in a mixing bowl except use only ½ can tomato sauce for the mixture. Mix all ingredients thoroughly. Spray nonstick baking sheet with butter spray. Shape turkey into balls and place on baking sheet. Top each meatball with a spoonful of remaining tomato sauce and additional sprinkle of Italian seasoning. Bake for 25 to 30 minutes or until done. Sprinkle with parmesan cheese, if desired. Cool. Store in airtight container, and refrigerate.

Crock Pot or slow cooker method: Thoroughly spray inside of Crock Pot with cooking spray. Place meatballs in Crock Pot and top each meatball with a spoonful of remaining tomato sauce and an additional sprinkle of Italian seasoning. Cook on low 5 to 6 hours or high 3 to 4 hours. Sprinkle with parmesan cheese, if desired. Cool. Store in airtight container, and refrigerate. Serve hot or cold.

Note: Double recipe above for larger batch.

Makes 4 servings

Dinner

Meatloaf

2 packages ground turkey breast (1 to 1.25 pounds)
1 packet meatloaf seasoning
1–4 oz can green chilies
1–4 oz can tomato sauce (divided) **or**
1–10 oz can diced tomatoes with green chiles
½ cup dry oatmeal
1 whole egg
2 tsp ground cumin
1 tsp garlic powder
1 tablespoon parsley flakes
Butter flavored cooking spray

Combine all ingredients in a large mixing bowl, except ½ can tomato sauce and mix thoroughly. Preheat oven to 375°. Spray nonstick loaf pan with butter spray and coat well. Place meatloaf mixture in loaf pan and smooth surface. Pour remaining ½ can tomato sauce over loaf and use a spoon to cover well. Sprinkle with additional parsley and garlic powder. Bake 55 to 60 minutes or until done.

Makes 6 to 8 servings

Honey Mustard Chicken

6 boneless, skinless chicken breasts
3/4 cup honey mustard dressing
1 tsp basil
1 tsp paprika
1 tsp dried parsley
Butter flavored cooking spray
Dash salt and pepper

Trim all excess fat from chicken breasts. Preheat oven to 350°. Sprinkle chicken breasts with salt and pepper to taste, and place in a 9x13 inch baking dish that has been coated with butter cooking spray. In a small bowl, combine the honey mustard dressing, basil, paprika, and parsley. Mix well. Pour half of this mixture over the chicken, and brush to cover. Bake in the preheated oven for 30 minutes. Turn chicken pieces over and brush with the remaining 1/2 of the honey mustard mixture. Bake for an additional 10 to 15 minutes, or until chicken is no longer pink and juices run clear. Let cool 10 minutes before serving.

Makes 6 servings

Teriyaki Turkey Steaks

1 package turkey breast steaks (approximately 4-5 steaks or 1 lb)
McCormick's Grill Mates Teriyaki Marinade

Cover steaks with 1/4 bottle of the marinade in airtight container and shake well to make sure all steaks are coated with marinade. Grill steaks approximately 6-7 minutes each side or until done.

Serve with 1/2 corn on the cob with *I Can't Believe its not Butter* spray, and fresh or grilled veggies.

Makes 4 to 5 servings

Meatball Soup

You may choose to use pre-made meatballs from the meatball sandwich recipe for this soup also.

4 cans low sodium beef broth
1 low sodium beef bouillon cube
1 cup diced celery
1 cup diced carrots

½ medium onion, sliced
3-4 small red potatoes, cubed

Meatballs:
2 packages ground turkey breast (1 to 1.25 pounds)
2 tbsp parsley flakes
2 tsp garlic powder
2 tsp onion powder
½ cup dry oatmeal
1 egg
1 tsp salt
1 tsp pepper

Combine all ingredients for meatballs and mix well. Shape into balls with hands. Spray inside of Crock Pot with nonstick cooking spray. Place meatballs in bottom of Crock Pot. Place all vegetables and beef bouillon cube on top of meatballs. Slowly add beef broth. Cover and cook on low 5 to 6 hours or high 3 to 4 hours. Serve with ½ cup cooked *No-Yolks* egg noodles, if desired.

Makes 6 to 8 servings

Vegetable and Chicken Bake

6–8 oz chicken breast
1 cup mushrooms
1 cup zucchini cut into ¼ inch slices
4 green onions, sliced
1 small Roma tomato
1 tbsp parsley
¼ tsp basil
¼ tsp garlic powder
Salt and pepper to taste

Preheat oven to 350°. Trim any excess fat from chicken. Place chicken in casserole dish and cover with vegetables and seasonings. Bake for 30 minutes or until chicken is no longer pink.

Makes 1 serving

Baked Fish in Foil

6–8 oz fish fillet (Cod, Halibut, Grouper, Orange Roughy, etc.)
½ small onion, sliced into rings
½ cup carrots, sliced
1 small Roma tomato, sliced
1 small red potato, cut into 1 inch cubes (optional)
2 tsp lemon juice
¼ tsp basil
¼ tsp garlic powder
¼ tsp dill
Salt and pepper to taste
Heavy duty aluminum foil

Wash fish fillet and pat dry. Place fillet on dull side of a sheet of aluminum foil. Coat with lemon juice, dill, basil and garlic powder. Place vegetables over fillet with tomatoes on the top. Sprinkle with salt and pepper and any extra seasonings. Fold the right and left side of the foil sheet over the top so that one piece is over the other. Fold the top and bottom ends neatly so that no juices will escape. Place seam side up in the oven and bake at 325° for 15 to 25 minutes or until fish flakes and potatoes are done.

Makes 1 serving

Turkey Chili

2 packages ground turkey breast (1 to 1.25 pound packages)
1–28 oz can chili beans
1–15 oz can kidney beans
1–28 oz can whole tomatoes
1–4 oz can green chilies
2 tsp garlic powder
2 tsp chili powder
2 tsp ground cumin

Place uncooked ground turkey in bottom of Crock Pot and use fork to coarsely separate meat. Sprinkle turkey with garlic powder and chili powder. Drain canned tomatoes and kidney beans. Empty all canned contents into Crock Pot over turkey meat. Combine all ingredients well. Set on low 5 to 6 hours or high 3 to 4 hours. Garnish with fat free sour cream when serving.

Makes 6 to 8 servings

Chicken Enchiladas

1–3 pound package boneless, skinless chicken breasts
1–36 count package corn tortillas
2–16 oz containers low fat ricotta cheese
2–4 oz cans green chilies
2–15 oz cans green chile enchilada sauce
2 tsp garlic powder
2 tsp ground cumin
Salt and pepper to taste
Butter flavored cooking spray

Trim all excess fat from chicken breasts. Place in Crock Pot and sprinkle with salt and pepper. Cook chicken on low 5 to 6 hours or high 3 to 4 hours. Place chicken (without juices) in a covered mixing bowl or storage container. Shred chicken with fork until finely shredded. Add ricotta cheese, green chiles, garlic powder, and cumin and combine all ingredients thoroughly. Spray a 9x13 inch baking dish with butter cooking spray. Place 2 to 3 small spoonfuls of chicken mixture in the center of a corn tortilla. Roll tortilla tightly and place seam side down in the baking dish. Repeat until you have 2 layers (top and bottom) in the baking dish. Pour both cans of the green chile enchilada sauce over the enchiladas. Bake at 375° for 25 to 30 minutes or until sauce is bubbly and top layer is slightly golden. Serve with fat free sour cream.

Optional cooking method for chicken: Bake chicken breasts on a nonstick baking sheet (sprayed with cooking spray) for 30 to 45 minutes, or until chicken is no longer pink in center. Transfer chicken breasts to mixing bowl and follow directions above.

Makes 18 servings

Burritos

1 package ground turkey breast (1 to 1.25 pounds)
1 packet burrito seasoning
1 package whole grain or fat free tortillas
1–14 oz can black beans, drained
1 Roma tomato, diced
Green chile salsa

In a nonstick skillet, brown turkey and follow directions on the back of the seasoning packet. Warm tortillas in the microwave. Place ¼ cup turkey mixture and 2 tablespoons black beans in the center of the tortilla. Roll and garnish the burrito with tomatoes, green chile salsa, and fat free sour cream, if desired.

Makes 4 to 6 servings

Hearty Stew

2 packages turkey breast steaks (1 to 1.25 pound packages)
1 packet beef stew seasoning
1 cup carrots, cut into bite sized pieces
1 cup celery, diced
3–4 red potatoes, cut into 1 inch cubes
1 small yellow onion, cut into 1 inch pieces
1 tsp garlic powder
1 tsp onion powder
1 tablespoon parsley flakes

Cut turkey breast steaks into 1 to 2 inch pieces. Place in bottom of Crock Pot. Add seasonings and vegetables. Add seasoning packet and follow directions on the back for the amount of water to add to the stew. Cook on low 5 to 6 hours or high 3 to 4 hours or until potatoes are done.

Makes 6 to 8 servings

Stroganoff

1 pound turkey breast steaks
1 (10 3/4-ounce) can 98% fat-free cream of mushroom soup, undiluted
1 tsp garlic powder
½ medium onion, chopped
½ cup sliced fresh mushrooms
1 tbsp parsley flakes
½ teaspoon Worcestershire sauce
½ cup fat free sour cream
Salt and pepper to taste
No Yolks egg noodles

Cook noodles according to package directions. Drain noodles and place back in saucepan to keep warm. Cut turkey breast steaks into 1 inch strips. Spray nonstick skillet with butter flavored cooking spray and cook turkey strips and onion over medium high heat until cooked through and slightly browned. Reduce heat to low and stir in mushroom soup, mushrooms, parsley, Worcestershire sauce, salt and pepper. Simmer until mushrooms are cooked through. Add sour cream and combine all ingredients well. Remove from heat and serve over cooked noodles.

Makes 4 servings

Side Dishes

Marinated Balsamic Vinaigrette Salad

3 Roma tomatoes, sliced
1 large cucumber, sliced
½ medium red onion, sliced into rings
2 cups green leaf lettuce or spinach leaves
1 cup red cabbage
½ cup balsamic vinaigrette dressing (see recipe)

Prepare salad dressing according to previous recipe. Wash and slice all vegetables. Place everything except lettuce or spinach in airtight storage container. Pour dressing over vegetables. Close lid tightly and shake well. Let chill 2 to 3 hours before serving. Serve over fresh lettuce or spinach greens.

Sweet Potatoes

1 medium sweet potato or yam
1 tsp pumpkin pie spice
2 tsp *Splenda*
Butter flavored cooking spray or *I Can't Believe its Not Butter* spray

Wash potato well. Place in microwave for 5 to 6 minutes on high power or until potato is done. Slice in half and slice top of potato open. Gently mash potato so that it stays inside the skin. Spray with butter spray to coat top. Add *Splenda* and pumpkin pie spice. Serve warm.

Sweet Potato Casserole

3 to 4 medium sweet potatoes or yams, washed, peeled and cut into 1 inch cubes
1 tablespoon pumpkin pie spice
1 to 2 tablespoons *Splenda*
Butter flavored cooking spray
¼ cup pecan halves (optional)

Spray inside of Crock Pot with cooking spray. Place potatoes inside. Sprinkle pumpkin pie spice and *Splenda* over sweet potatoes. Spray additional cooking spray over potatoes to coat well. Mix thoroughly so that all potato pieces are coated well. Turn on low 5 to 6 hours or high 3 to 4 hours. Serve warm with 1 to 2 tablespoons pecan halves and additional spices, if desired.

Seasoned Steamed Veggies

1 to 1½ cups fresh mixed vegetables such as (broccoli, carrots, cauliflower, zucchini, etc.)
¼ tsp oregano
¼ tsp garlic powder
¼ tsp basil
¼ tsp parsley flakes
Salt and pepper to taste
Butter flavored cooking spray or *I Can't Believe its Not Butter* spray

Wash and cut fresh vegetables. Mix seasonings well in a separate bowl. Steam vegetables until softened. Spray vegetables lightly with butter spray. Sprinkle seasoning mixture over vegetables and mix well. Serve warm.

Zucchini with Onions

2 to 3 medium zucchinis, peeled
1 small to medium yellow onion, sliced into rings
1 tbsp parsley flakes
1 tsp garlic powder
Salt and pepper to taste
Butter flavored cooking spray
Parmesan cheese sprinkle (optional)

Peel zucchinis and cut into halves. Cut halves into halves again until you have ½ inch strips or julienne strips. Place zucchini in large, airtight container. Slice onions into rings and place in container. Coat top layer of zucchini and onions with cooking spray. Sprinkle seasonings over the top and cover with lid. Shake vigorously to coat all pieces. Spray nonstick pan with additional cooking spray. Sauté zucchini and onions until zucchini is soft and onions are transparent and slightly golden. Serve with 1 teaspoon parmesan cheese and salt and pepper to taste.

Creamy Veggie Dip

1 packet *Hidden Valley Ranch Buttermilk Recipe Dressing*
16 oz fat free sour cream
¼ cup fat free mayonnaise
2 green onions, finely chopped
1 tsp parsley

Place all ingredients, except onions and parsley, in a food processor and blend until smooth. Place in airtight container and mix in onion and parsley. Chill 2 to 3 hours before serving. Serve with fresh cut vegetables such as cucumbers, broccoli, cauliflower, carrots, and celery.

Zesty sour cream

1–6 oz container light plain yogurt **or**
1–8 oz container fat free sour cream
¼ tsp chili powder
¼ tsp ground cumin

Combine ingredients well in yogurt container. Chill before serving.

Lemonade or Limeade

Juice of 6 lemons or limes
1 cup *Splenda* sweetener
2 to 2 ½ quarts ice water

Slice lemons in half and squeeze juice thoroughly from each half into a bowl. Strain lemon juice into a large pitcher. Add ice water and *Splenda* and mix well. Note: Start with 2 quarts water and add more for desired taste.

Tips & Tricks

♦ *For zesty eggs, add a tablespoon of salsa (red or green) on top.*
♦ *Sprinkle red wine vinegar or seasoned rice vinegar on salads for a change.*
♦ *Use Dijon and honey mustard dressings as alternative veggie dips.*
♦ *Slice whole grain tortillas into triangles and bake until crisp and dip with salsa for a snack.*

14-Day Menu Plan

Week 1

Monday

Breakfast
1 egg - ¼ cup egg whites
½ cup cooked oatmeal with *Splenda*
3 slices turkey bacon

Mid a.m.
6 oz light yogurt
2 to 3 hardboiled egg whites

Lunch
Grilled chicken breast
½ **sweet potato**
½ can green beans

Mid pm
Fruit & cottage cheese delight

Dinner
Turkey burger
½ cup cooked carrots
½ can green beans

Optional
½ cup **fruit salad**

Tuesday

Breakfast
Veggie omelet
3 slices turkey bacon

Mid am
½ cup cottage cheese with *Splenda*
½ cup pears

Lunch
Creamy chicken salad
Sliced cucumber with **balsamic dressing**
1 slice whole grain bread

Mid pm
½ **turkey burger**
1 tablespoon ketchup
1 cup mixed raw veggies

Dinner
Chicken soup

Optional
½ **turkey burger**
½ medium cucumber sliced with lite salt & pepper

Wednesday

Breakfast
1 egg + ¼ cup egg whites
3 slices turkey bacon

Mid am
Fruit & cottage cheese delight

Lunch
Meatball sandwich
½ cup **marinated salad**

Mid pm
6 oz light yogurt
2-3 hardboiled egg whites

Dinner
Turkey burritos
½ cup **seasoned rice**

Optional
Chicken salad
1 whole grain tortilla

Thursday

Breakfast
1 egg + ¼ cup egg whites
3 slices turkey bacon

Mid am
½ cup **Fruit salad**

Lunch
Turkey Burger
½ cup **sweet potato casserole**
Green salad

Mid pm
Fruit & cottage cheese delight

Dinner
Teriyaki turkey steaks
1 cup steamed broccoli and carrots

Optional
Chicken soup

Friday

Breakfast
1 egg + ¼ cup egg whites
½ cup oatmeal with berries and *Splenda*
2 slices turkey bacon

Mid am
Smoothie

Lunch
Turkey chili

Mid pm
Tuna salad
1 whole wheat tortilla

Dinner
Meatball soup

Optional
½ cup **fruit salad**

Saturday

Breakfast
Omelet
3 slices turkey bacon

Mid am
Fruit and cottage cheese delight

Lunch
Italian meatballs
½ cup marinated salad

Mid pm
Smoothie

Dinner
Baked fish in foil

Optional
Turkey jerky

Sunday—Free Day!

Week 2

Monday

Breakfast
1 egg + ¼ cup egg whites
Oatmeal pancake
3 slices turkey bacon

Mid am
Smoothie

Lunch
Honey mustard chicken sandwich
½ **sweet potato**
½ cup **seasoned veggies**

Mid pm
3-4 **Italian meatballs**

Dinner
Meatloaf
½ cup **marinated salad**
½ **sweet potato**

Optional
½ cup **fruit salad**

Tuesday

Breakfast
Veggie omelet
3 slices turkey bacon

Mid am
½ cup cottage cheese with *Splenda*
½ cup pears

Lunch
Grilled chicken salad

Mid pm
Turkey jerky
1 cup mixed raw veggies

Dinner
Chicken enchiladas

Optional
Fruit parfait

Wednesday

Breakfast
1 egg + ¼ cup egg whites
3 slices turkey bacon

Mid am
Fruit and cottage cheese delight

Lunch
Meatball sandwich
½ cup **marinated salad**

Mid pm
6 oz light yogurt
2-3 hardboiled egg whites

Dinner
Stroganoff
Green salad

Optional
Chicken salad
1 whole grain tortilla

Thursday

<u>Breakfast</u>
1 egg + ¼ cup egg whites
3 slices turkey bacon

<u>Mid am</u>
Fruit salad

<u>Lunch</u>
Turkey burger
½ cup **sweet potato casserole**
Green salad

<u>Mid pm</u>
Fruit and cottage cheese delight

<u>Dinner</u>
Teriyaki turkey steaks
1 cup steamed broccoli and carrots

<u>Optional</u>
Chicken soup

Friday

<u>Breakfast</u>
1 egg + ¼ cup egg whites
½ cup oatmeal with berries and *Splenda*
2 slices turkey bacon

<u>Mid am</u>
Smoothie

<u>Lunch</u>
Turkey chili

<u>Mid pm</u>
Tuna salad
1 whole wheat tortilla

<u>Dinner</u>
Meatball soup

<u>Optional</u>
½ cup **fruit salad**

Saturday

<u>*Breakfast*</u>
Omelet
3 slices turkey bacon

<u>*Mid am*</u>
Fruit and cottage cheese delight

<u>*Lunch*</u>
Italian meatballs
½ cup **marinated salad**

<u>*Mid pm*</u>
Smoothie

<u>*Dinner*</u>
Baked fish in foil

<u>*Optional*</u>
Turkey jerky

Sunday—Free Day!

Chapter 6

The Fitness Plan

Why the Weights Help You Lose Weight

Now that you have an understanding of the importance of nutrition, let's discuss the significance of resistance training with weight loss. It doesn't matter if you have 10, 30, 50, 100 or more pounds to lose; you need to start resistance training to see optimal results. My goal is to totally change your body's resting metabolic rate, and turn you into a fat burning machine! The best, most effective way to do that is to continue being consistent with the nutrition program and incorporate a weight training regimen. Resistance training is the *only* effective way to lose body fat, reshape your body, and kick your metabolism into high gear.

The reason why the weights work is that an increase in your lean muscle mass, from moderate to intense weight training, signals your body to burn more calories to sustain its muscle mass. This calorie burning frenzy never stops, as long as you continue to weight train. In fact, it gets better and better every year with consistency. Muscle cells require a larger amount of energy (in the form of calories) to sustain them. Therefore, calories that would normally be consumed and then stored, are immediately expended, eliminating all storage possibilities. However, this is only the case when you are consuming good, quality, whole foods, that your body and muscles prefer. The byproduct of weight training results in a slimmer, firmer, and shapelier physique, and an increase in resting metabolic rate also. Weight training alone produces these dramatic results, *not* cardiovascular exercise.

It is really rewarding to see your body change with weight training. Probably the most exciting benefit from weight training is the physique transformation. Your body will begin changing its composition of body fat as muscle mass increases. You will lose inches as well as body fat weight. Here is a general physique transformation timeline and the changes you should expect to see and feel:

Physique Transformation Timeline—What to Expect

Week 1–Week 2

This is the introductory period when you are becoming familiar with the weights and the exercises given. You will also begin to learn and understand the importance of training *intensity* and muscle *endurance* that is needed to make considerable progress. You should expect to feel a moderate amount of muscle soreness which is normal following your weight training routine. This will be further discussed in the next section.

You should take a *before* picture for your reference the day before you start. Even though the thought of getting in front of a camera makes you squirm, you need to do this. This is truly the best way to really see your progress. Believe it or not, you will become accustomed to your new physique and forget about the old one. So make it a priority, after all this is an investment in *you*.

Week 3–Week 4

During this phase of your program, you should be comfortable with most of the exercises and beginning to increase your weights gradually. Initially, you will feel lots of different changes happening in the muscles, i.e., muscle firmness. This change begins the day you start weight training and significantly increases thereafter. Your overall feeling of wellness will dramatically improve. You will also notice that clothes are fitting better in certain areas like the waist and/or hips.

It is important to note that when your body begins to metabolize body fat, your body fat loss will not be evenly distributed. In other words, the body usually begins to shed excess fat in the places you would least like to see it gone. Don't be discouraged by this, in fact, you need to take heed during this phase. It is during this unique time that you need to remain focused on consistency to continue to see results. Your body will continue to lose body fat at a steady pace and begin to snowball until your body eventually gives in and sheds those last remaining pounds. You should expect to see changes during this phase, even if they may seem small. Remember that these pounds didn't just appear overnight, and they won't disappear overnight either.

Week 5 and on...

Consistency is the main ingredient to seeing better results each *week*. Yes! You can expect to continue seeing changes week by week. From this point on, you should be making your workouts a routine part of your life. You should always challenge yourself, even if it's just a small increase in weight or performing a few more repetitions. Your workout routines should become more advanced and your endurance level will dramatically improve with each session. The sky is the limit here, so work hard and you will be rewarded!

Not only will your physical appearance noticeably change, but your overall health will benefit greatly from weight training. Most notably, bone density will increase. This is the best way to increase your bone density naturally. Basically, the increased resistance that is being applied to the muscles also applies to the bones. Tendons and ligaments that make up the joints will increase in strength, flexibility, functionality, and range of motion. There will also be less overall pressure applied to the joints as the muscles become stronger, thereby eliminating overuse.

Other significant benefits of weight training include lower blood pressure, lower resting heart rate, decreased blood cholesterol, and decreased risk of cancer, diabetes, heart disease and other ailments.

As you can see, the benefits of weight training are endless. It is the best kept secret on defying the aging process. The greatest part is that no matter what age you start, you will reap the benefits with consistency. Basically, this means that a 60-year-old woman that has been weight training for 10 years can dramatically look and feel better than a 30-year-old woman who is sedentary. The proof is in the pudding so don't put this off anymore. Be the best that you can be at *any* age!

Work out at Home or the Gym—No Excuses!

Basic Definitions

Repetition(s) Amount of repeated, controlled movements of an exercise that is performed.

Set(s) Number of repetitions of an exercise done in sequence.

Super Set An exercise that is performed back to back with another exercise with minimal or no rest time in between.

Drop Set A set that is performed at a heavier weight, then the weight is reduced by a certain amount, and a subsequent set is performed. Weight may continue to be reduced subsequent more times to complete a drop set.

Concentric A contraction, in which a muscle exerts force, shortens and overcomes a resistance; also referred to as the *positive* aspect of an exercise.

Eccentric A contraction, in which a muscle exerts force, lengthens and overcomes a resistance; also referred to as the *negative* aspect of an exercise.

Lateral Anatomical term meaning away from the midline of the body; pertaining to the side.

Anterior Anatomical term meaning toward the front.

The *Burn* A build up of lactic acid characterized by a warm or hot sensation in a muscle as a result of anaerobic training.

Lactic Acid A waste product of anaerobic production known to cause localized muscle fatigue or *the burn*.

Delayed Onset Muscle Soreness (DOMS) Muscle soreness that occurs 24 to 48 hours after intense exercise. Typically associated with eccentric muscle contraction, and thought to be the result of microscopic tears in the muscle or connective tissue.

Muscle Endurance The capacity of a muscle to exert force repeatedly against a resistance, or to hold a fixed or static contraction over time.

Muscle Failure When muscle contraction, either positive or negative, fails to continue as a result of intense physical effort.

Momentum Increasing the speed of the exercise to allow for faster repetitions.

Reverse Pyramid Opposite of the traditional pyramid training technique. Heaviest set is performed after the warm up and then weight is reduced for subsequent sets.

Testosterone The hormone that is directly responsible for the production of muscle cells found in both men and women.

Before we dive right into the workouts, I want to explain a few important things you should know and expect during and after your training sessions whether you are training at home or the gym.

The 3 Types of Pain

There are 3 types of pain that you need to understand because they are all *very* different.

1. The Burn

The burn has been around for a long time. It has been made popular by the eighties style aerobics classes where the instructor would shout out, "Go for the burn!" This is that dreaded, uncomfortable, warm (or hot), nagging pain in the muscle(s) that usually disappears after you stop doing the exercise. Basically, the *burn* is a build up of **lactic acid**, the byproduct of muscle contractions, which is released into the blood stream.

Lactic acid is a waste product of anaerobic energy that produces muscle fatigue. This is usually a harmless sort of pain, if you can bear through it. What's more important is that when your muscles are burning, you have the opportunity to increase the speed of your results by how much you can *push* through the burn. This time is a true test of your **muscle endurance**, and the best way to increase your endurance is to try to do a few more **repetitions**.

2. Delayed Onset Muscle Soreness

Delayed onset muscle soreness or DOMS is characterized by the soreness that you experience 24 to 48 hours following a workout. This pain should be moderate in intensity and can usually be alleviated by gentle stretching, ibuprofen, or hot pack, if necessary. This type of pain is harmless and usually goes away in 1-5 days, depending on your exercise intensity. Know that though the initial soreness may be overwhelming, your body will adapt quickly and the muscles will not be nearly as sore by your next workout. You will find that it will be more challenging to become sore after each workout if you are consistent.

Also note that soreness is not necessarily the sign of a good workout. Your muscle endurance will increase greatly with consistency and even though you had an intense workout, you may not experience any soreness at all.

3. Sharp Pain

This last type of pain is characterized by sharp, nagging, pulling, or twisting sensations. If any of these apply, immediately *stop* doing the exercise! Don't try to push through this pain because you will only injury yourself more. This pain is sometimes felt in the joints or in a muscle. Most often poor technique or overuse is to blame which we will discuss in the next section. Listen to your body and recognize what feels right and what feels wrong.

Anaerobic vs. Aerobic Training

There are two different types of training that produce entirely different results and require different sources of energy. Aerobic basically means; with, or in the presence of oxygen. Aerobic activities can be low to moderate type activities like swimming, power walking, jogging, and bicycle riding. When training aerobically, the body recruits glucose, in the presence of oxygen, as its primary source for energy production. This glucose is metabolized by the body through a pathway know as glycolysis, or the breaking of glucose.

Anaerobic means the opposite; without the presence of oxygen; not requiring oxygen. The anaerobic metabolic pathway still uses glucose for energy production, but produces lactic acid as a byproduct. Anaerobic activities include weight training, sprinting, or any activity where the intensity level is high. Anaerobic glycolysis is also referred to as the lactic acid system. The anaerobic system can be done in short bursts while the aerobic system can be done over a period of time.

Importance of Training Intensity and Good Technique

Training intensity is the amount of effort, mentally and physically, that you invest in each workout session. Training intensity relates to quality, not quantity. It is that key moment when you feel like giving up because of muscle fatigue and burn, that you push yourself a little harder. Your training intensity level can make all the difference in the world if you really want to see good results. If you are distracted or trying to rush through your workouts, you will not benefit from the time spent. Make it worthwhile and push yourself a little harder each time. Here are some tips to help you improve your training intensity level.

1. Listen to music. Find motivating music that makes you feel like moving! Music helps you stay focused on the exercise at hand and eliminates outside distractions.

2. Inhale on the negative (downward) motion of the exercise and exhale on the positive (upward) motion of the exercise. This increase in oxygen intake helps you get those last few reps. Remember to never hold your breath. Always breathe!

3. Work out with a partner. Having a friend work out with you is a great way to motivate each other. Make sure your partner *spots* or assists you when you are getting close to **muscle failure**.

4. Incorporate **super sets** and **drop sets** in your routine. Super sets are exercises done back to back with very little rest time; <10 seconds. Drop sets are done by immediately *dropping* or *lowering* the weight 10-20 lbs, depending on the exercise, after each heavier set. Rest time is also very minimal; <10 seconds. Both of these training techniques will help to increase the training intensity level for optimal results.

5. Incorporate **holds** and **pulses** during and after your sets. Holds and pulses can be done anytime in your training routine. They are more intense if saved for the end of a set. Holds should be 5 to 10 seconds. Pulses should consist of a smaller, controlled movement, usually at the top of the motion. Always keep pulses smooth and controlled and eliminate all **momentum**. Just when you think you can't do anymore, do a few holds and a few pulses.

6. Try not to focus on counting repetitions. Focus on the movement. Make sure you are in proper form and not using any momentum. Counting also limits you from working harder. Instead, do reps until you are feeling like you *can't* do one more, and then count 5 more repetitions. This will greatly increase your intensity level and results!

Intensity in your workout routines is paramount to your fitness success. Without the right amount of intensity it could quite possibly take you twice as long, if not longer, to see the same amount of progress. If you are just starting out, expect some periods of fatigue and exhaustion. You need to develop muscle endurance, so try to stay at a fairly intense level of training initially. Rest times should be longer during your first few weeks, so don't try to overexert yourself. Listen to your body and progress gradually.

Good technique or *form* is also a key for great results. Technique refers to how different aspects of your body are in relation to the amount of weight and exercise being performed. With poor technique you are more likely to sustain an injury. An example of this would be doing bicep curls and hyperextending your back (leaning back excessively) to help get the weights up. Not only are you not even helping the biceps, but you are encouraging a nagging back injury. I will give you reminders in the exercise descriptions about proper form with each exercise. Here are some things to remember about proper form in general:

1. Never hyperextend the back by leaning back as far as you can to get the weights up. If you feel yourself starting to do this in the beginning of the exercise, chances are the weight is too heavy.

2. Keep your knees slightly bent at all times in every exercise. Whether you are standing, sitting, or lying down, knees should be slightly bent or *soft* at all times. *Never* lock out your knees.

3. Keep your shoulders back. Don't allow yourself to slouch forward. Keep your shoulders in alignment with your spine.

4. Keep all movements, especially with weights, smooth and controlled. Don't use momentum to try to get done faster, you will only be wasting valuable time and encouraging an injury. Slower movements utilize muscle fibers to their maximum abilities. Proper breathing is also helpful when trying to slow down your movements.

5. Focus on your form. Good form can make all the difference in the world! Smooth, controlled movements can dramatically increase the intensity of any exercise. So don't opt for more weight until you have mastered the form of the exercise.

The Rule of 10

The Rule of 10 is something that we developed that keeps you in the best training zone. I want you to stop focusing on counting reps. Counting is not only distracting, but often times the intensity level desired is never attained because you are only focusing on your goal of *x* number of reps instead of the exercise. You should, however, be in the 8 to 10 repetition range, as this is the most effective for strengthening and shaping muscles.

You will always start with a warm up set and get about 10 to 15 reps. The warm up should be somewhat challenging, but not overly intense. Remember, this is just the warm up set. Then I want you to increase the total weight by 10 pounds. This will be your *heavy* set. I want you focus on your form here, not just flinging the weights around. Now, if your form is compromised, stop immediately and drop down 5 pounds into a range where you are challenged and keeping proper form. You will then proceed to drop the weight in smaller increments for each remaining set.

The secret here is that if you can do 10 reps fairly easily, meaning that you could easily get 5 or more, you need to increase the total weight by 10 pounds. This is how you can determine if you are training intensely enough. If you can't reach 8 reps, you're weights are probably too heavy, and if you can get more than 10, you're weights are too light.

The Reverse Pyramid Technique

The Reverse Pyramid Technique is the exact opposite of the traditional style of weight training. The Pyramid Technique is when you start with a warm up set then gradually increase the weight for each consecutive set with your heaviest weight being used for the last set. What's wrong with this type of training is that you are not getting the most benefit for your time. Basically, you are slowly fatiguing the muscles until the last set where you are to totally expend all remaining energy and intensity. The previous sets were not maximizing muscle endurance capacity and are essentially wasted.

The Reverse Pyramid is the opposite. Like the traditional method, a warm up set is recommended. After warm up, increase the weight by 5, 10, or 15 pounds to your *max* weight. This increase in weight will depend on the exercise at hand. The max weight should be a weight that is challenging but does not compromise your form or posture. You should also be getting between 8 to10 reps in this set. Remember, this should be *challenging*.

You will then take a 30 second rest and proceed to drop down in weight in small increments for each consecutive set. You may choose to do a drop set where your rest is shorter, around 10 seconds, and you drop the weight by 10 to 20 pounds depending on the exercise. Either way, the heavier set should be done relatively early on in the exercise. You will continue to drop down until your final set. You should expect to feel a significant amount of burn here, so *try, try, try,* to push through it!

The reason why the reverse pyramid is so effective is that the heavier set of the exercise is intended to **build** the muscle by increasing the muscle's density and size. Ladies, pay special attention here. It is a myth that you will *bulk* or get bigger in size with moderate resistance training. In fact, the opposite happens. You will find a more slender, firmer, and stronger physique as a result of your hard work.

The hormone **testosterone** is directly responsible for increasing muscle size and growth. So for us ladies, this doesn't amount to much because we don't produce a great deal of this hormone. Men, however, will produce much faster muscle gains because of the inherent testosterone they produce. It is also important to note that your increase in muscle mass will not result in an increase in scale weight. This is a big misconception. It has been reported that is takes an entire year of intense, consistent resistance training for a women to put on 5 pounds of muscle! For men it's about 10 to pounds. So, you should definitely see the scale, inches, dress or pant size, and body fat go down as you put on lean muscle mass.

The lighter sets of the exercise focus a little more on muscle *shape* and definition. It makes sense to do your heavier set first because this is when you have the most strength and endurance. The lighter sets should be done as you begin to fatigue, but you are still able to get more reps with better form because the weight is lighter. This combination has proven to be extremely effective for seeing considerable muscle development in a much shorter amount of time.

Variation of Exercises

The key to seeing better results week by week, month by month, and year by year, is to make sure you have a good variation of exercises in your workout routine. Not only will this eliminate the boredom factor, but the body will respond quickly by being *shocked.* This shock or variation can be large or small, like increasing the weight by 10 pounds, or even changing the hand placement with the weights, or changing the angle of motion. Either way, make sure you are *challenging* yourself in your routines rather than just going through the motions. It is important to keep the body guessing, never allowing it to predict what is coming next. The end result is a stronger, sculpted body in the shortest amount of time possible. We will discuss the variations that you should use with each exercise in the next section.

How Long and How Often Should You Workout?

Session length of time and workout frequency will have a dramatic effect on your results. But how much is really necessary? The Surgeon General has revised the recommendations for daily aerobic type activity to 30 minutes every day. While this may seem like a lot of time, it really isn't. If you really want to see and feel changes, you're going to have to dedicate the time to it. My recommendations are outlined below. You can do either three 1 hour training sessions, or a six day routine where you are training a half hour per day. These sessions will give you an intense workout in a short amount of time.

The idea here is to train every muscle group intensely one time per week. This is by far the most effective training method to see great results. Circuit training, where you train multiple muscle groups every session, is the least effective when trying to produce a greater increase in lean muscle mass. This type of training is better for improving overall endurance, not strength, and increasing heart rate for a cardio effect. I want you to focus on good, quality weight training sessions, not short, circuit training sessions.

It is possible to overtrain your muscles, which will hinder your progress. When you exceed 1 ½ hours of intense resistance training, your body is beginning to fatigue and will refuel itself by breaking down muscle protein to make glucose for quick energy. Not only will you feel completely wiped out afterwards, but you will not reap the benefits of your session. Don't overdo it. Stay within the 1 hour zone and work hard to complete your routine.

Cardio Plan

The purpose of my cardio plan is to emphasize cardiovascular health and a temporary increase in calorie burning while keeping your appetite stabilized (not elevated). Note that the cardio plan is completely optional. You can get the *same* effects with a moderate to intense resistance training session. Make sure that if you do the cardio plan that you limit your session time to 30 minutes, 3 times per week.

The cardio exercises should be low to moderate in intensity and should consist of things you enjoy doing like walking, hiking, bike riding, etc. Also, find some good music to listen to during your session. This makes a big difference in maintaining your intensity level and motivation. If you choose to monitor heart rate as a way to determine intensity, use the following formula:

220-Age = Max HR

220-40 = 180 beat per minute (bpm)

The goal is to stay somewhere between 50-70% of your maximum heart rate.

.50 x 180 = 90 bpm

.70 x 180 = 126 bpm

The *talk test* is a simpler way to determine cardio training intensity. If you can carry on a conversation during your training with relative ease, meaning, you are not completely struggling to get the words out, you are in the right training zone.

The Best of the Best Exercises
Complete Home Workout

Below are two different training schedules that you can choose depending on your schedule. Note that these schedules apply to your home or gym workouts.

Suggested 3-Day Schedule

Monday—Arms (Biceps & Triceps)

Wednesday—Legs

Friday—Shoulders, Chest, & Back

Session Length

1 hour

-or-

Suggested 6-Day Schedule

Monday—Biceps
Tuesday—Triceps
Wednesday—Legs
Thursday—Shoulders
Friday—Chest
Saturday—Back

<u>*Session Length*</u>

30 minutes

<u>*Everyday Exercises—3-5 days per week (for both schedules):*</u>

Abs

Buns and Inner/Outer thighs (alternate each day)

<u>*Session length*</u>

10-15 minutes

<u>*Cardio Plan (Optional)*</u>

No more than 3 days per week, 30 minute sessions.

Activities: Power walking (indoors or outdoors), bike riding, swimming, or any other low to moderate intensity cardiovascular activity.

Let's Get Started!

Abdominals
When training abs, always start with the lower abdominals and work your way up to the upper abdominals.

Beginner/Intermediate
Do 2 to 3 sets each exercise, 10 to 15 repetitions or until complete muscle failure. Try to get at least 5 to 10 pulses (very small, slower movement), and one 5-10 second hold at the end of each set.

Advanced
Do 3 to 4 sets of each exercise until muscle failure. Be sure to include pulses and holds in every set as you approach muscle failure.

Lower Abdominals

Reverse Curls

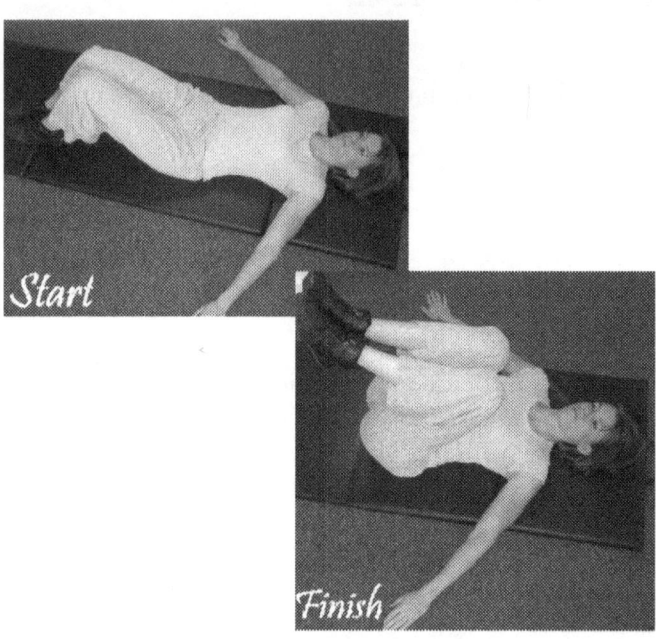

Starting position:
Lying with your back flat on the mat and arms extended outward, palms facing down. Emphasis is on keeping the low back down (not arched), and abdominals contracted.

Tip: Try not to use any momentum to lift the rear off the mat, use the abs.

The movement:
Keep the knees together and bring them toward your chest. Lift the rear slightly off floor and contract the lower abs. Return to starting position except keep heels right above the floor. Repeat movement.

Heel Raises

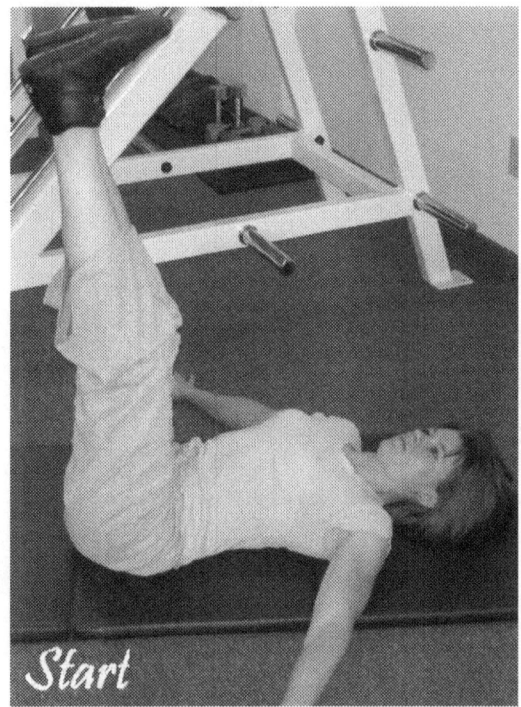

Starting position:
Keep your lower back into the mat and legs straight up. Emphasis is on pressing the low back down into the mat and contracting the abdominals.

The movement:
Keeping the legs straight and together with heels facing the ceiling, gently lift the rear up off the floor, contracting the lower abs. Lower the rear back down for a slight pause and begin the next repetition.

Tip: Keep the legs straight and try not to use momentum.

Bicycles

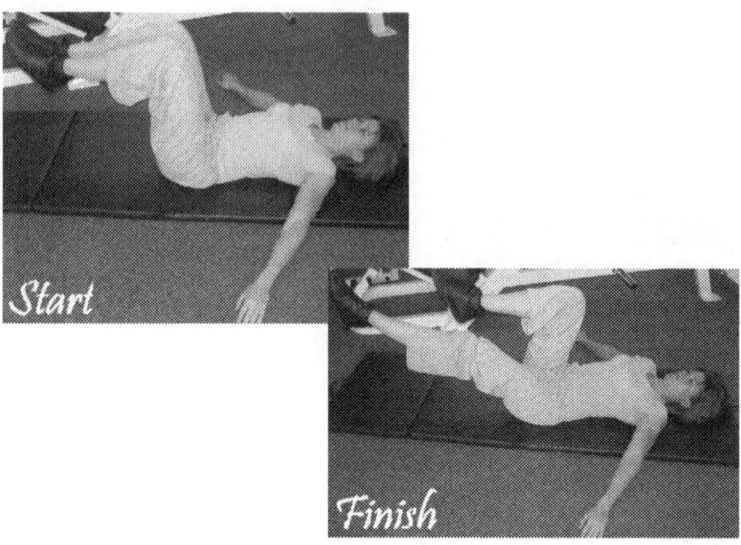

Starting position:
Lower back down and knees up.

The movement:
Slowly extend one leg out to an almost straight position. Bring the leg back in and alternate. Emphasis on lower back pressed down into the mat.

Tip: If you feel your back arching as you fully extend the leg, decrease your range of motion.

Straight Leg Raises

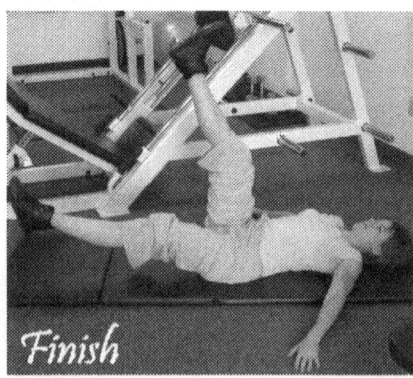

Starting position:
Lower back down and legs straight up.

The movement:
Slowly lower one leg down just above the mat. Bring the leg back to starting position and alternate.

Tip: If you feel your back arching as the leg gets closer to the floor, decrease your range of motion.

Upper Abdominals

The Crunch

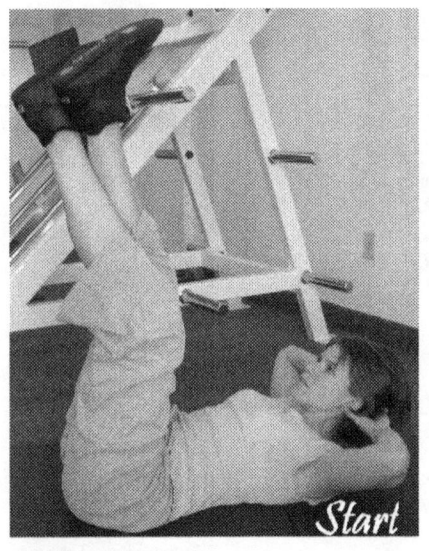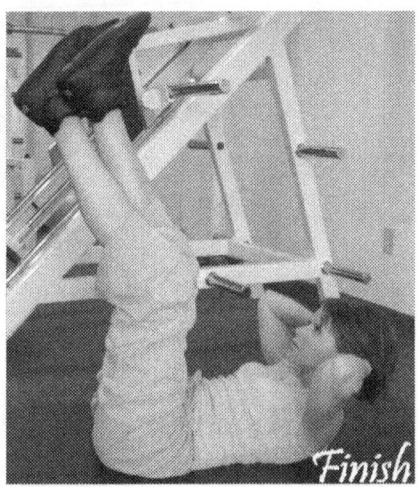

Starting position:
Hands gently supporting the back of the head. Elbows stay outward. Eyes are drawn upwards toward the ceiling. Legs straight up, crossed at the ankles.

The movement:
Using the upper abs, crunch up to your highest point. Come back down just above the floor and repeat.

Tip: Think of trying to get your shoulder blades as far off the floor as possible. This will allow you to use your abs instead of pulling on your head with your hands.

Tip: If your legs get tired, you may bend at the knees.

Obliques (Side Abdominals)

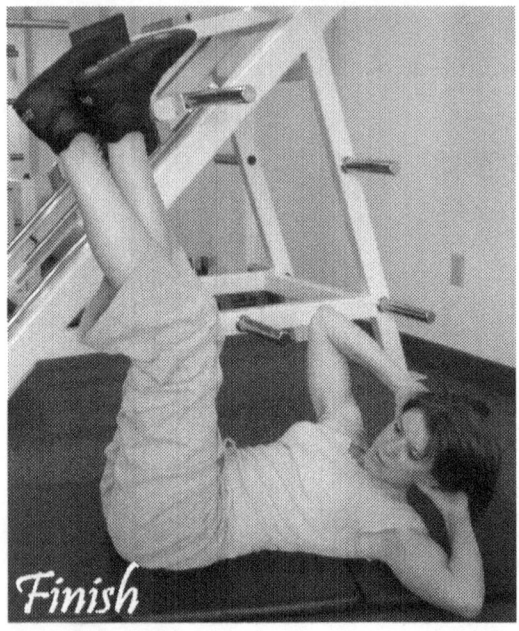

Starting position:
Same as the crunch.

The movement:
Crunch up and over toward the side of the body. Return to starting position, just above the mat and alternate.

Tip: Think of leaving the floor with the shoulder, rather than the elbow.

Tip: Keep movements smooth and controlled, don't force or pull on the head and neck. Don't try to touch the elbow to the knee.

Advanced Abdominal Exercises

Reverse Curl
Contract upper abs and hold, keeping the upper abs stationary. Keeping knees together, raise knees toward chest, contracting both upper and lower abs. Slowly lower the heels above the mat and repeat.

Heel Raises
Contract upper abs and hold. Raise legs straight up and keep together. Lift the rear off the floor while keeping the upper abs stationary.

Bicycles
Contract the upper abs and hold. Slowly extend one leg at a time and alternate while keeping the upper abs stationary.

Alternating Oblique/Bicycle Combo

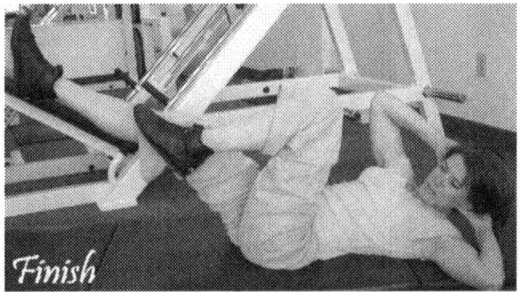

Perform bicycles as normal. Incorporate alternating oblique crunches with alternating legs.

Crunches

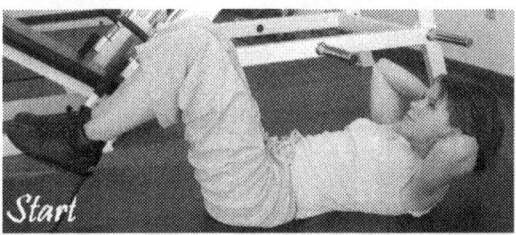

Raise heels just above the floor and push slightly outward. Crunch the upper body while maintaining leg position.

Obliques
Same position as crunches, but alternate side to side.

Floor Work

Buns

Lying Pelvic Tilt

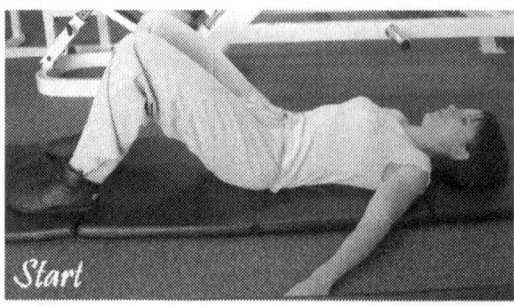

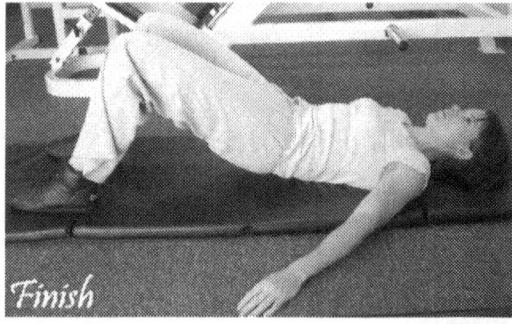

Starting position:
Lying flat on your back, place feet about shoulder width apart. Press lower back down and place hands outwards, palms facing downward.

The movement:
Tilt the pelvis forward (toward you) and lift hips upwards. Contract and squeeze the buns. Return to starting position just above the mat and repeat. Include pulses and holds toward the end of each set.

Tip: This should be a small range of motion, if you are going too high, focus on pressing your lower back down toward the mat.

Tip: Don't release the contraction at the bottom of the movement, but rather maintain the contraction and squeeze up a little harder each time.

Lying Rear Leg Extension

Starting Position:
Lie facedown on the mat. Head, neck, and shoulders remain down.

The movement:
Keeping the leg straight (knee soft), lift the leg up to its highest point, contract the buns, and return to starting position just above the mat.

Tip: Make sure your hips stay on the mat and upper body stays down to protect your lower back.

Tip: To isolate the buns more, decrease your range of motion to a pulse, and decrease your speed.

Inner Thighs

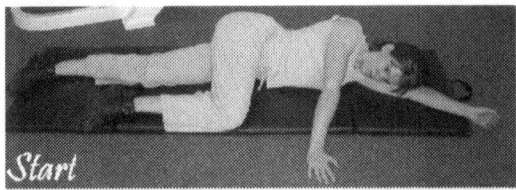

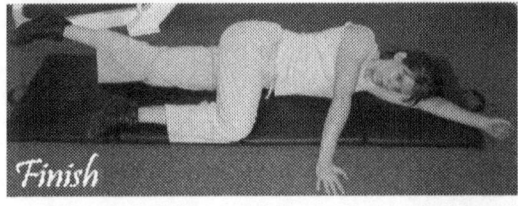

Starting position:
Lying on your side, place the top knee and foot on the floor and extend the bottom leg. Top arm is reaching forward to maintain position.

The movement:
Slowly raise bottom leg upwards, contracting the inner thigh muscle. Return to starting position, just above the mat and repeat.

Tip: This is a small movement so focus on slow, controlled movements.

Include pulses and holds as well as these various combinations:

Heel pushes: Slightly bend at the knee and then extend the leg back out, while keeping the leg off the floor.

Circles: Keeping the leg up, make slow circles with the leg. Try not to make the circles with just the foot. Try clockwise and counterclockwise movements.

Advanced Variation:
Rise up onto your elbow. Bend the top leg at the knee and place top foot flat behind bottom leg. Extend bottom leg and lift to contract the inner thigh.

Include previous movements and also:

Sweeps: Keeping the leg up, slowly extend away from the body or sweeping out contracting the inner thigh. Slowly return to starting position.

Knee-Ins: Keeping the leg up, slowly bring the knee toward the chest and slowly extend back out to straighten the leg and contracting the inner thigh.

<u>Outer Thighs</u>

Straight Leg Lifts

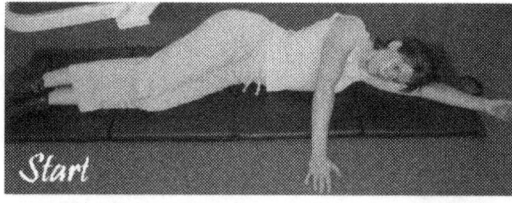

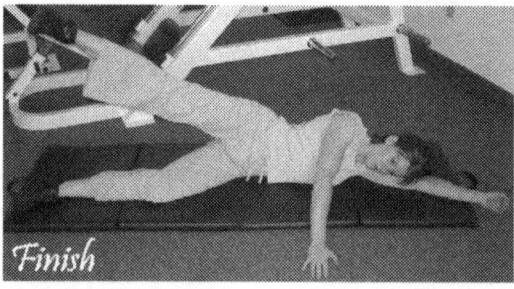

Starting position:
Lie on your side so that you are completely on the bottom hip. Keep top leg straight and slightly bend the bottom leg for comfort and reach forward with the top arm to maintain position.

The movement:
Raise top leg up 45 degrees and lower just above the floor and repeat.

Tip: Make sure that you are keeping in the correct position by reach forward with the top arm. Don't let yourself lean back as you fatigue.

Tip: Don't raise the leg past 45 degrees. Keep the movements slow and controlled.

Include these variations at the end of the movement:

Heel pushes: Keeping the leg at the 45 degree angle, slightly bend at the knee and extend the leg back out to straight position.

Pulses: Keep the leg at the top of the movement and slowly pulse up and down, maintaining a smaller range of motion.

Circles: Same as inner thighs. Make a small, circular movement with the working leg.

Advanced Variations (for all outer thigh exercises):

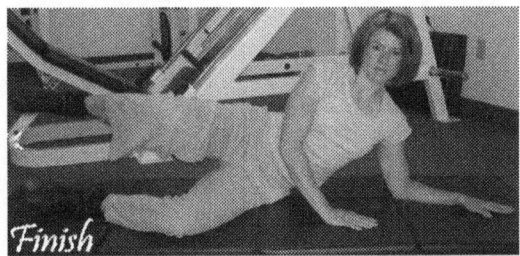

Rise up onto the elbow so that you are comfortably on top of the bottom hip. Perform movements as instructed. Include pulses and holds at the end of every set. Make sure you are going to complete muscle failure!

45 Degree Push Outs

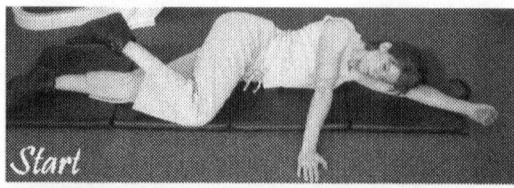

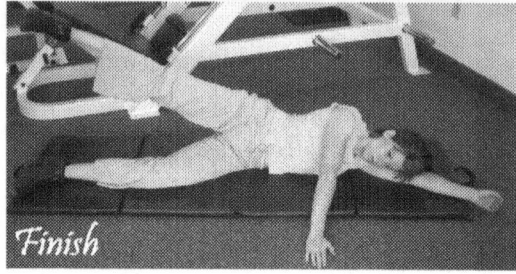

Starting position:
Lie on your side so that you are completely on the bottom hip. Keep top and bottom legs slightly bent and stacked on top of each other. Reach forward with top arm to maintain position.

The movement:
Bring the top knee to the floor and angle the heel upward 45 degrees. Extend the leg out maintaining the 45 degree angle.

Tip: Don't extend the working leg behind the bottom leg, keep legs aligned.

Tip: Make sure you bring the knee back to the floor to touch briefly for complete range of motion.

Bent Knee Raises

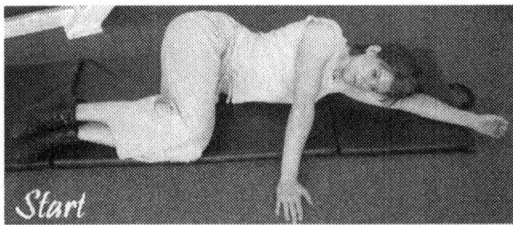

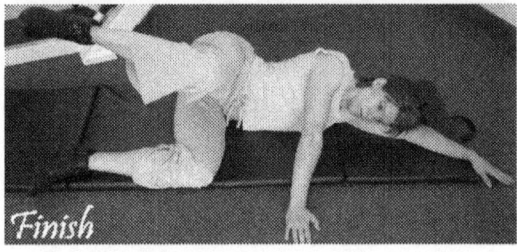

Starting position:
Lie on your side so that you are completely on the bottom hip. Bring both knees toward the chest to make a 90 degree angle and keep legs stacked on top of each other. Reach forward with top arm to maintain position.

The movement:
Keeping this position, raise the top leg up to a halfway point and lower down just before the resting point.

Tip: Don't raise the leg too high here. Keep a small, controlled movement.

Arms

<u>Biceps (front of the arm)</u>

Bicep Curls—Dumbbells

Hold dumbbells with palms facing forward. Keep elbows stationary and *locked* into the sides of the body. Bend at the elbows and curl upwards, contracting the biceps.

Tip: Keep the knees slightly bent and shoulders back to maintain proper form. If you are arching your back to try to get the weights up, the weight is too heavy.

Isolation Curls

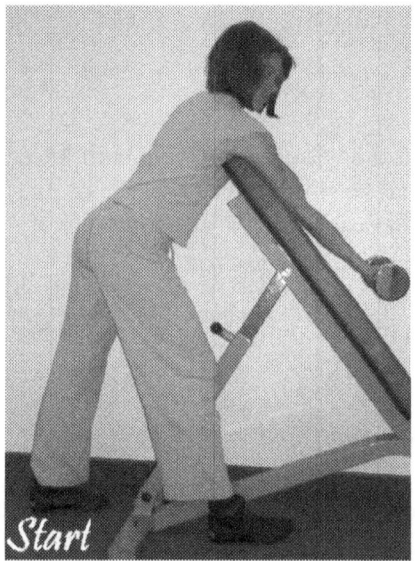

Using an incline bench, place upper arm completely flat against bench. Extend arm almost straight and then contract the bicep to bring the weight up.

Biceps Curls–Curl bar

Place hands comfortably in the curved part of the bar. Keep elbows stationary and locked to the sides of the body. Curl the bar upwards, contracting the biceps.

Tip: Keep the knees slightly bent and shoulders back. If you are arching your back to help get the weight up, the weight is too heavy.

21's

This is the same movement and technique as dumbbell bicep curls. First, do 7 full range of motion repetitions and hold at the top. Next, do 7 halfway down and back to the top and hold at the halfway position. Then, finish with 7 down (arms extended) and halfway up. Finish with a ten second hold in the halfway position.

Triceps (back of the arm)

Lying Triceps Extensions or "Skull Crushers"

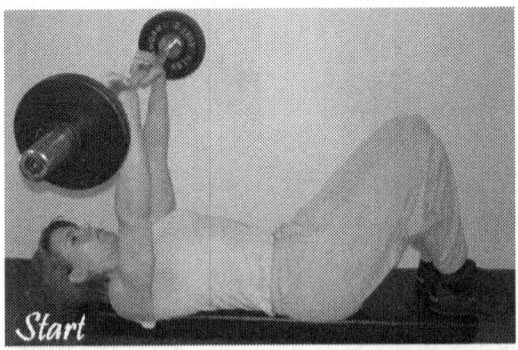

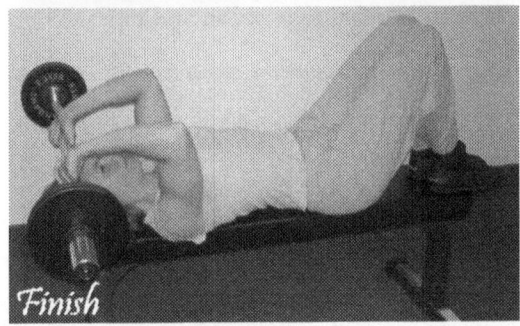

Lie flat on the bench. With a curl or straight bar extend arms so that they are straight over the body, placing your hands in the closest curved parts of the bar or fairly close together with the straight bar. Keep your elbows forward and stationary. Slowly lower the bar just above the forehead and push back up to starting position.

Tip: As you fatigue make sure your elbows don't bend outward.

Variation:
Use dumbbells instead of the bar. Hold onto ends of dumbbells and keep dumbbells separated. Alternate lowering arms toward the end of the set.

One Arm Extensions

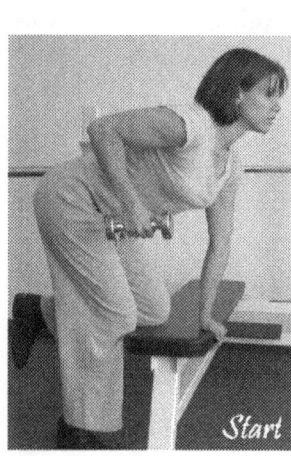 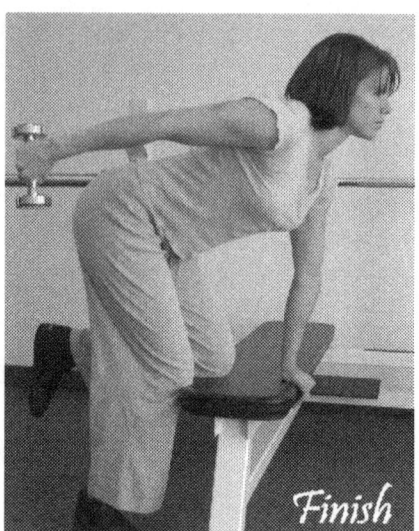

Using a flat bench, place one knee (closest to the bench) on the bench and opposite leg slightly bent. Bend over keeping your back flat. Bring the elbow up and lock into the side of the body. Keep the upper arm stationary and extend the lower arm up to contract the triceps. Return to starting position and repeat.

Tip: Don't try to lock out the elbow or raise your arm above the shoulder.

Triangle Pushups

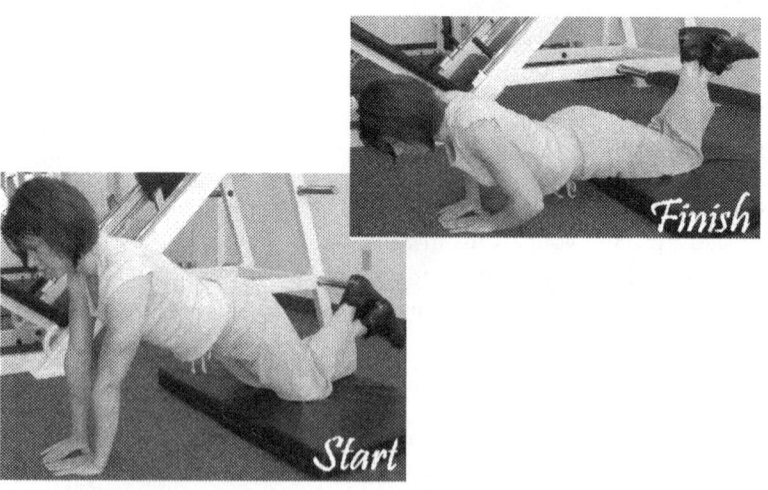

Using a mat to support your knees, extend your body forward and arms slightly forward supporting the body. Make a triangle with your hands by angling both hands inwards. Slowly lower your upper body and bend at the elbows as you come down towards the floor. Push back up to starting position.

Tip: Don't lock out the elbows at the top of the movement.

Advanced variation: Extend legs out to a regular pushup position on the toes.

Dips

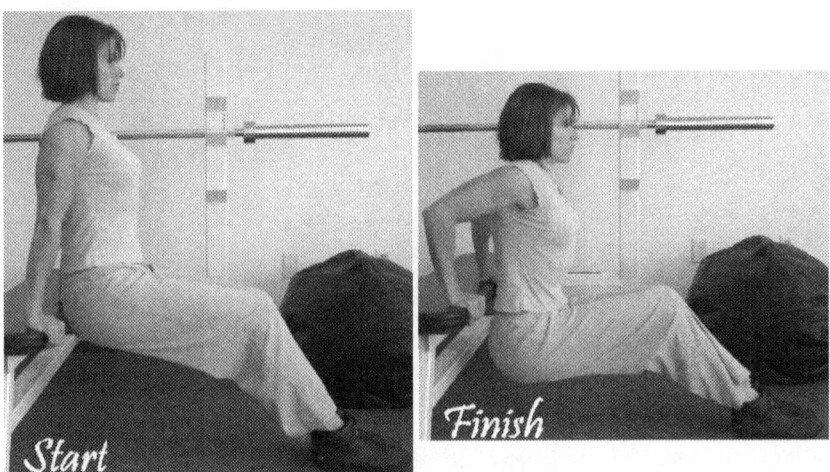

Using a flat bench, sturdy chair, or coffee table, place palms on the edge and grip the underside gently with your fingers. Position your backside so that it is fairly close to the edge of the bench and move your legs out in front of you, bending at the knees. Slowly lower yourself towards the floor so that your upper arms are parallel to the floor and push back up to starting position.

Tip: Don't move out too far away from the bench as this will stress the shoulders and wrists.

Advanced variation: Extend legs out straight instead of bent.

Legs

Thighs, Buns & Hips

Stationary Lunges

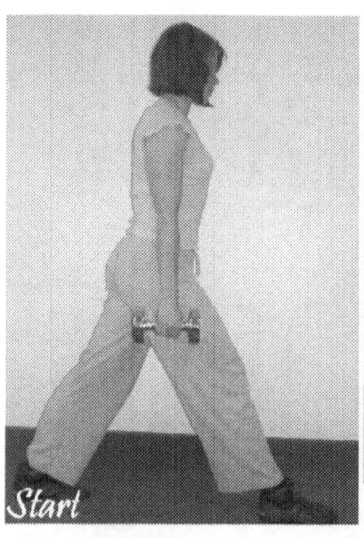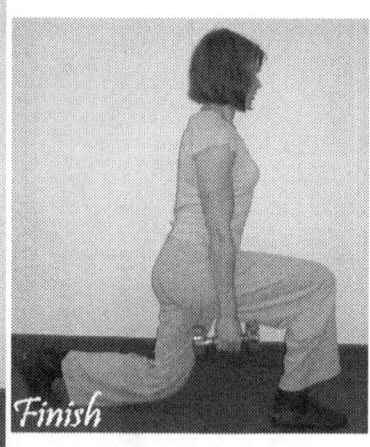

Starting with feet together, step forward with one leg and lower the back knee towards the floor. Keep the upper body upright and use your arms for balance. Rise back up by straightening the legs and repeat.

Tip: Keep the front knee in line with the front toe. Don't let the knee go over the toe.

Tip: Make sure that the back knee bends right away otherwise you will feel a strain in the back thigh muscle.

Advanced variation for all movements: Hold dumbbells in the hands while performing the exercise.

Alternating Lunges

This is the same as stationary lunges except push back with front leg to return to starting position and alternate legs.

Tip: Make sure you take a wide enough step forward to prevent the front knee from going over the toe.

Alternating Reverse Lunges

Instead of stepping forward with the lunging leg, take a wide step backwards. Immediately bend at both the front and back knees, bring the back knee towards the floor. Use the front leg to then pull the back leg back up to standing. Repeat.

Tip: Keep the body upright as you perform this exercise and try not to lean too far forward for balance.

Walking Lunges

Same as alternating lunges but instead push forward with front leg and bring both legs together back to standing position. Alternate legs so that you are moving forward for each repetition.

Tip: Do these slowly as you will have better balance and form.

Advanced variation: Instead of bringing both legs together after each lunge, step forward into the next lunge.

Wall Squats

Place an exercise ball against the wall and position yourself so that your low/mid back is pressed firmly against the ball and place your feet out two steps out in front of you. Slowly lower down towards the floor as if you were going to sit down in a chair. Push back up through the heels to starting position. Repeat.

Tip: Keep the knees soft at the top of the movement—don't lock them out.

Tip: Don't go below 90 degrees with the legs as this will stress the knees.

Advanced variation: Hold dumbbells at your side while performing the movement.

Inner Thigh Squats

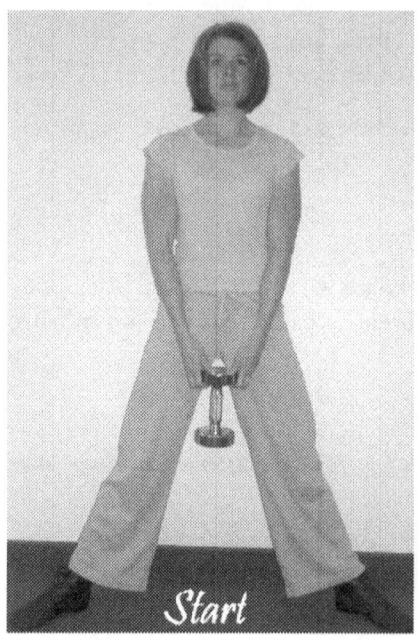
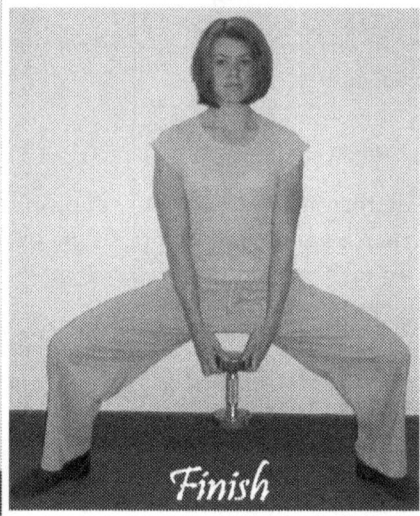

Stand with feet wider than shoulder width apart and toes angled outwards. Lower your body down so that the thighs are parallel to the floor. Push slowly up to starting position. Repeat.

Tip: Keep upper body upright and don't use your hands to help push yourself up.

Tip: Keep the knees slightly bent at the top of the movement to increase tension in the thighs.

Advanced variation: Hold dumbbell while performing the movement. Also try raising one heel off the floor while performing the exercise for half the reps and alternate. This puts additional emphasis on the thighs.

Hamstrings, Buns & Calves

Dead Lifts

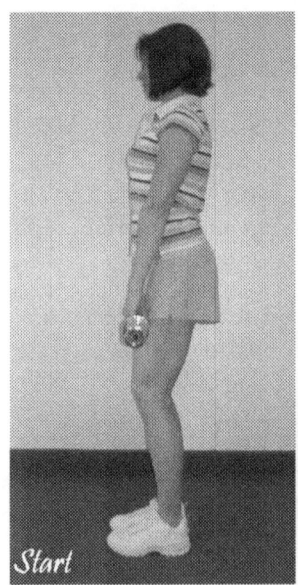
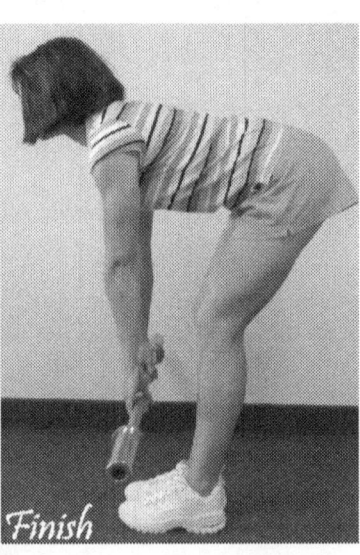

Holding dumbbells or a weighted bar, slowly lower down, keeping your back very flat, head looking forward and knees slightly bent. Lower down until you feel a deep stretch in the back of the legs. Return to starting position keeping the back flat and shoulders relaxed.

Tip: Think of pushing the buns out first as you lower your upper body.

Tip: Don't lock out the knees; keep them soft or slightly bent at all times.

Tip: Hold the bar with your arms straight; don't try to raise the bar up with your shoulders.

Standing Hamstring Curls

Hold onto a chair or sturdy object. Stand with feet together and knees slightly bent. Keep the knees together and slowly curl your heel toward the buns contracting the back of the leg. Lower to a halfway position and repeat movement.

Tip: Make sure the supporting leg or standing leg is slightly bent and relaxed.

Tip: Keep your body properly aligned—shoulders back and stand straight. Also keep a comfortable grip on the chair but not a death grip!

Advanced variations: Add ankle weights to this exercise up to 10 pounds. Also include these variations:

Pulses & Holds: Toward the end of the set or until you reach muscle failure, pulse the leg up slow and controlled and hold ten seconds to further increase muscle failure.

Heel Pushes: Same starting position. Keep the lower leg parallel to the floor or halfway up. Slowly push the heel back to feel a more intense contraction in the hamstring. Return to starting position and repeat.

Lying Hamstring Curls

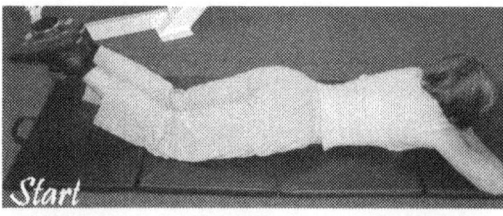

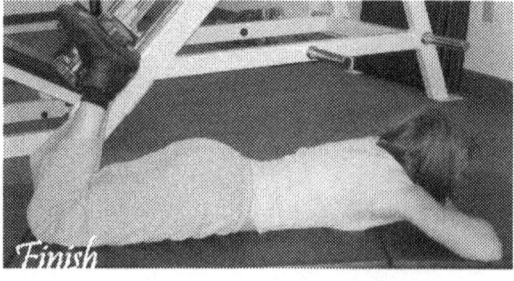

On your knees, place a dumbbell securely in between both feet. Lie face down on a mat. Start with knees bent and back of the legs contracted at the top. Slowly lower the dumbbell towards the floor, hold for a brief moment and return to starting position.

Tip: Keep your hips down and back flat. If you find yourself arching your back, decrease the amount of weight.

Advanced variation: Perform this movement face down on a flat bench.

Hamstring Squeeze

Lie flat on a mat and position your heels on the edge of a flat bench or coffee table. There should be a 90 degree angle at the knees. Keeping your legs and feet together, push up through your heels and lift your hips slightly off the floor, squeezing through the hamstrings. Hold for a moment at the top of the movement and repeat.

Tip: Make sure that you are not coming too high off the floor. Focus on keeping the lower back down. Keep the legs together and focus on pushing through the heels at all times.

Standing Calf Raises

Place the front of the feet on the edge of a stair and lightly hold onto the rail for support. Rise up onto the top of your toes, contracting the calf muscles. Lower down so that your heels go below the edge of the stair and contract the calf muscles again by raising to the top. Repeat.

Advanced variation: Do a set with feet angled outward (heels together), and feet angled inward (heels apart).

Shoulders

Military Press

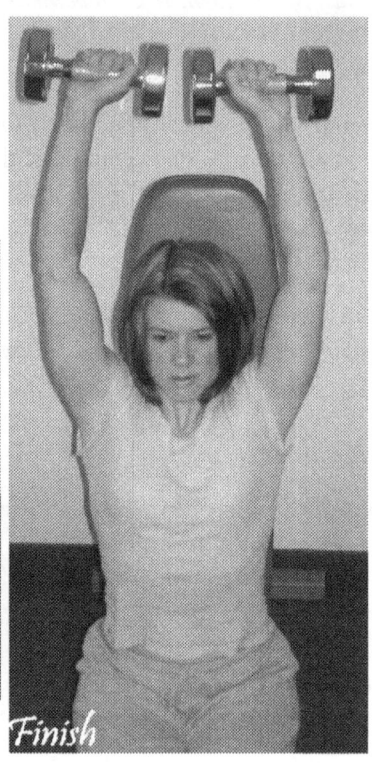

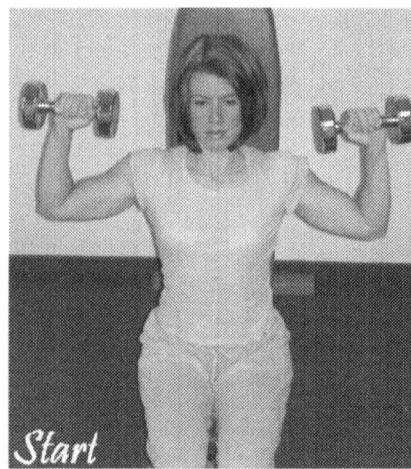

Place the incline bench in the upright position or use a sturdy, well padded chair. Hold dumbbells, palms facing forward, at shoulder level. Push dumbbells directly overhead so that the arms are almost straight and dumbbell ends are almost together. Slowly lower back to starting position. Repeat.

Tip: Keep a slight arch in the lower back for support. If you feel that you are arching your back too much then decrease the weight.

Upright Rows

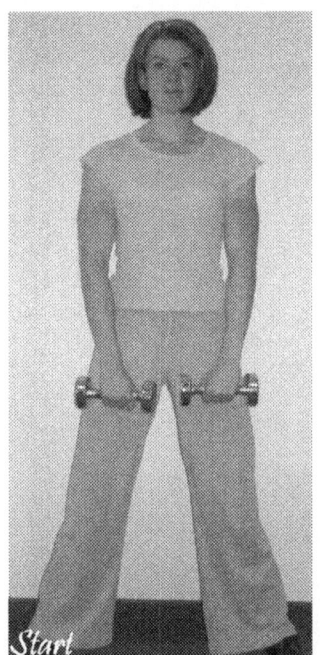 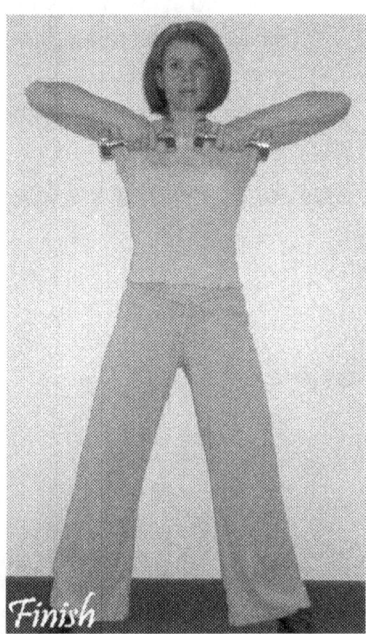

Keeping the knees slightly bent, hold a weighted bar or dumbbells in front and raise the elbows up, bringing the weight up towards the chin. Slowly lower back to starting position. Repeat.

Tip: Think of leading with the elbows. Elbows should be the highest (above the shoulders) at the top of the movement.

Tip: There should be no momentum here. Keep the movement smooth and controlled.

Front Raises

Keeping the knees slightly bent and arms fairly straight (elbows soft), raise dumbbells in front of the body, up to shoulder level with palms facing the floor. Slowly lower back to starting position. Repeat.

Tip: Don't swing the weights up, keep a controlled movement.

Tip: Don't raise dumbbells past shoulder level.

Advanced variation: Lower the weights halfway down and back up into the next repetition.

Side Raises

Keeping the knees slightly bent and arms fairly straight (elbows soft), raise dumbbells out to the sides of the body up to shoulder level, with palms facing the floor. Slowly return to the starting position. Repeat.

Tip: Don't raise the weights past shoulder level.

Advanced variation: Stop halfway and raise back up.

Rear Shoulder Raises

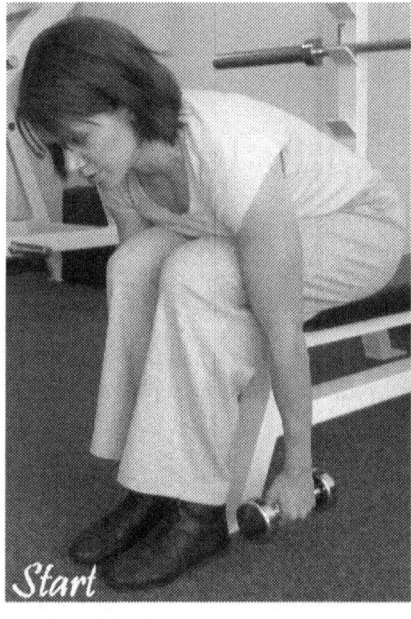
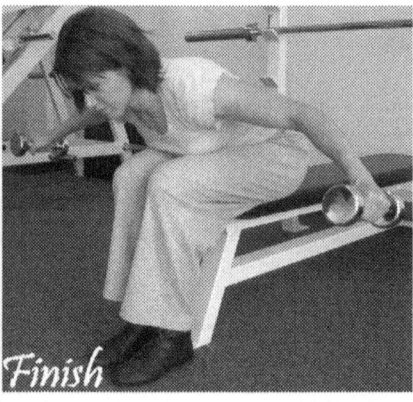

Sit with knees bent and lean forward keeping the back flat. Raise dumbbells up to shoulder level with palms facing the floor. Return to starting position and repeat.

Tip: Keep a flat back to ensure proper form.

Tip: Don't swing the weights. Keep a controlled movement. If you are using momentum, decrease the weight.

Chest

Flat Dumbbell Press

Using a flat bench, push dumbbells up directly over the center of the chest and turn the dumbbell ends inward. Slowly bend at the elbows, bringing the weights down to chest level. Push back up to starting position.

Tip: Think of pushing through the chest on the way up rather than the arms.

Tip: Keep your lower back down on the bench, if your back is extremely arched, the weights are too heavy. You may place your feet on the bench for support.

Variation: Perform this exercise on an incline bench.

Incline Bench Flys

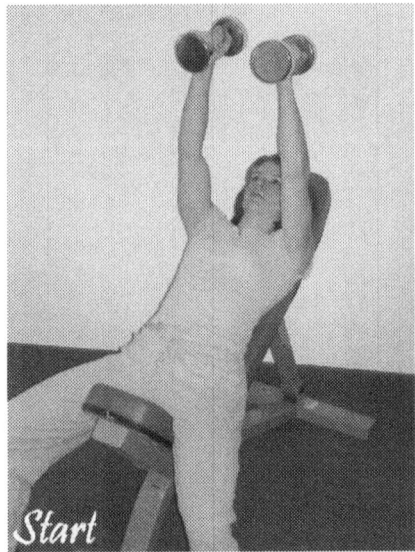 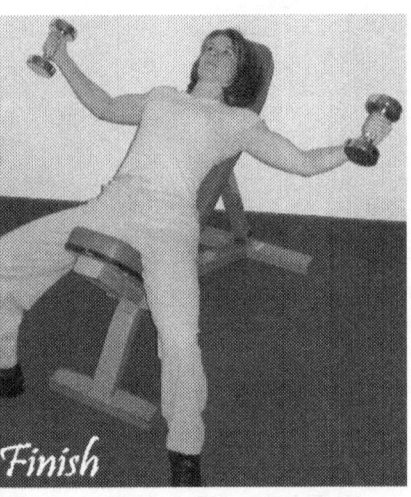

Start by pushing the arms up together keeping palms facing forward. Slowly lower the arms out to the sides keeping a slight bend in the elbow. Return to starting position and repeat.

Tip: Try not to go down too far. Lower the weights to a point where you feel a good stretch and bring the arms back together.

Tip: Keep a slow, controlled movement and try to use the chest to help pull the weights together.

Variation: These can be done on the flat bench also.

Pushups

Start by placing a mat under the knees for support. Extend your body in front of the mat so that you are completely straight, i.e., no arched or slouched back. Place your hands a little wider than shoulder width apart. Slowly lower the chest down towards the floor and push back up to starting position. Repeat.

Advanced variation: Perform pushups on the toes instead of the knees.

Back

One Arm Rows

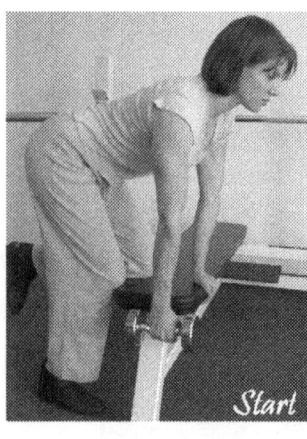 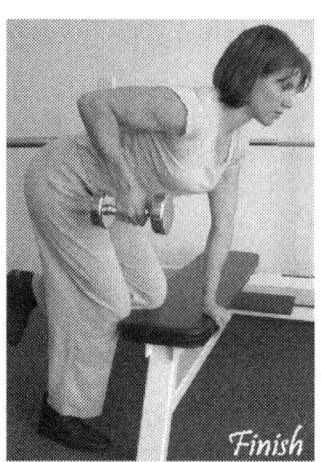

Using a flat bench, place one knee and hand (closest to the bench) on the bench and opposite leg slightly bent. Bend over keeping your back flat. Holding a dumbbell, extend opposite arm toward the floor. Raise the arm up, bending at the elbow and keeping the arm close to the body. Contract the mid back at the top of the movement. Slowly lower back down to starting position and repeat.

Tip: Keep the back very flat during this exercise.

Tip: Concentrate on the top of the movement and give an additional squeeze in the mid back.

Complete Gym Workout

Arms

Biceps

Preacher Curls

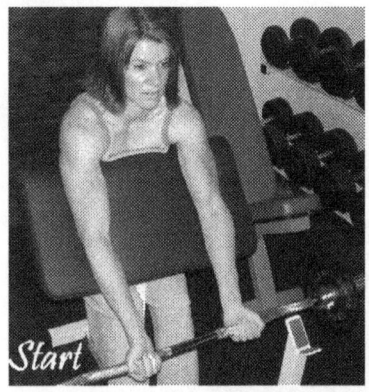 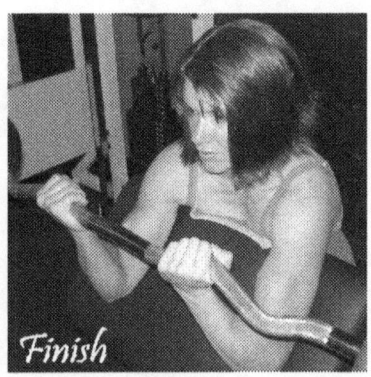

Place your upper arms against the pad leaning forward slightly. Comfortably grip the bar and lower almost to the point of complete extension in the arms. Bring the weight back to the top of the movement, contracting the biceps. Repeat.

Tip: Make sure that your upper arms are completely pressed against the pad.

Cable Curls

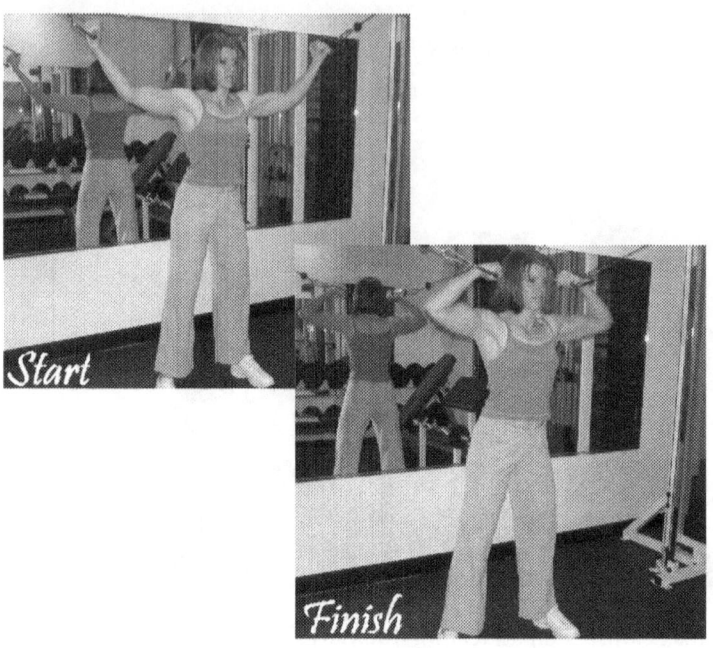

Standing centered at the cable machine with knees slightly bent, bring the handles all the way inward toward the ears, contracting the biceps. Slowly extend outward and repeat.

Tip: Keep the arms parallel to the floor and elbows back. If this is difficult to do, decrease the weight.

Advanced variation: Perform the exercise one arm at a time and hold the support handle on the opposite side of the machine.

One Arm Cable Curls

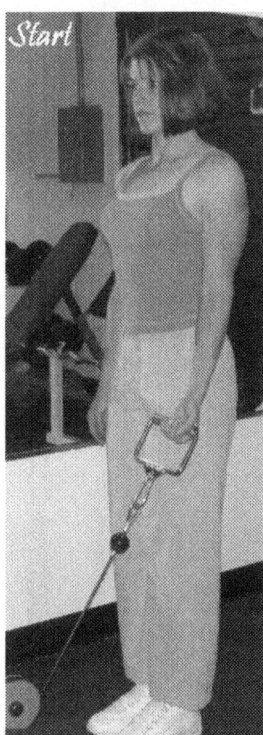 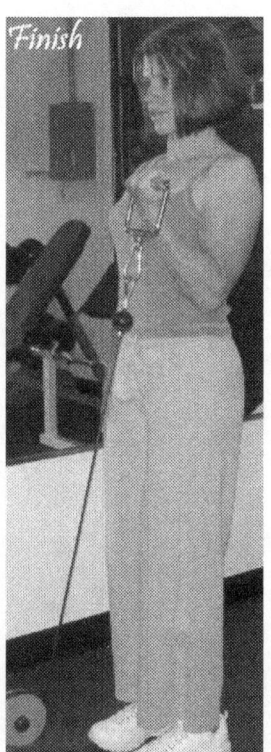

Standing with knees slightly bent and working elbow locked into the side of the body, bring the handle toward the shoulder, contracting the bicep. Slowly lower down and repeat.

Tip: If you find yourself arching your back to help get the weight up, decrease weight and keep the back neutral.

Triceps

Overhead extensions

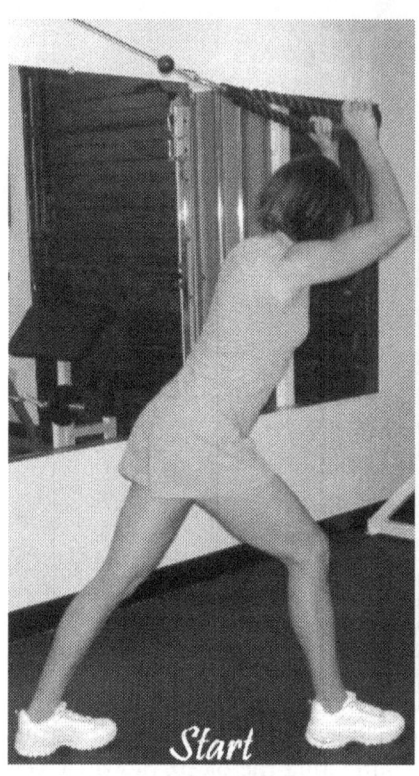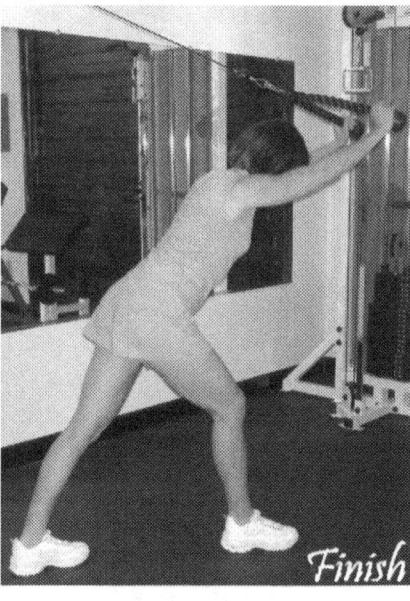

Use the rope attachment and position cable at the highest position. Turn around, and take a step forward. Position the upper arms so that they are parallel to the floor and keep them stationary. Extend forearms outward, contracting the triceps. Slowly lower the weight back, keeping the upper arms stationary, and repeat.

Tip: There should be no movement in the upper arms. Use the forearms and bend at the elbow.

Tip: Keep your back flat and avoid using any momentum.

Triceps Pushdowns

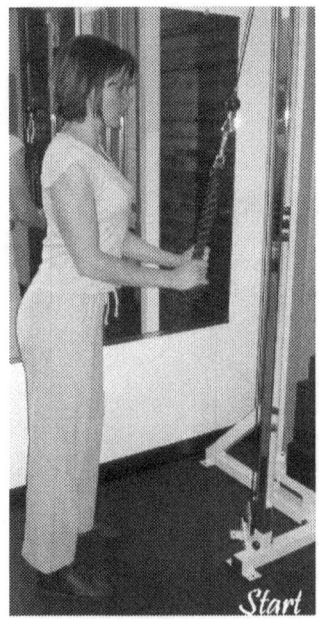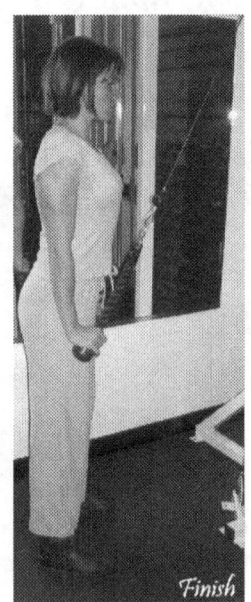

Stand with knees slightly bent. Comfortably grip the rubber ends of the rope attachment. Position your elbows so that they are locked into the sides of the body. Extend the arms down, taking the rope ends slightly outward at the bottom of the movement. Come back up to a halfway point and repeat movement.

Tip: Make sure the arms don't come up past the halfway point as this will take the emphasis off the triceps.

Variations: Use the straight bar attachment and do:

Close Grip: Overhand grip, hands close together.
Reverse Grip: Underhand grip, hands on the ends of the bar.

One Arm Extensions

Using the single handle attachment, take an underhand grip. Position the elbow so that it is locked into the side of the body. Extend the working arm all the way down to straighten, contracting in the triceps. Come back up to the halfway point and repeat.

Tip: As you fatigue, use the nonworking arm for assistance.

Legs
Thighs, Buns & Hips

Leg Press

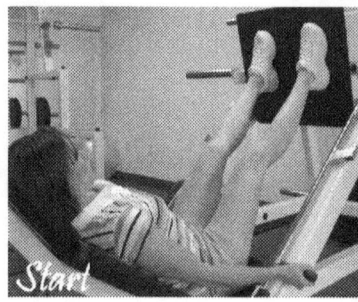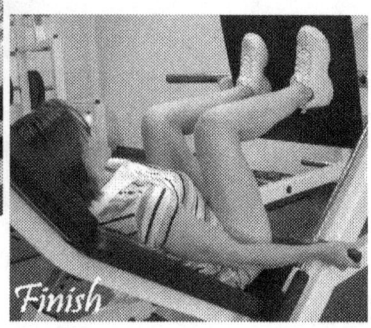

Place feet shoulder width apart. Slowly lower the platform down, maintaining contact with the heels on the platform. Push back up through the heels to starting position, keeping the knees soft. Repeat.

Tip: If you feel your buns lifting off the seat at the bottom of the movement, decrease your range of motion.

Tip: Don't let your legs touch your chest to try to come down lower. Keep the knees above the chest and focus on keeping your heels on the platform.

Leg Extensions

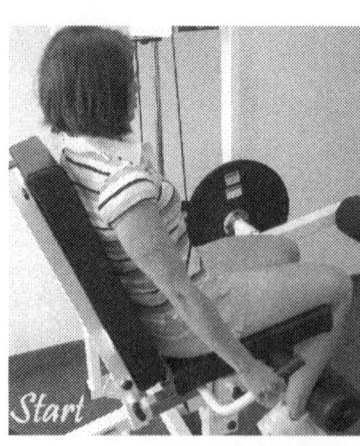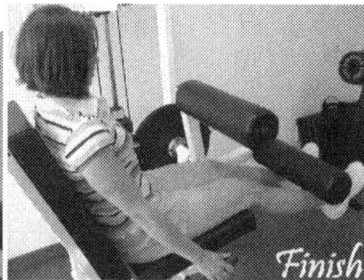

Sit comfortably with your back supported. Place feet under bottom pad so that pad is just above the feet. Slowly extend the legs outward, but do not lock out the knees. Come to a position just below complete leg extension. Hold for a moment, and return to starting position, but do not release the weight. Repeat.

Tip: Think of contracting the muscles in the thigh as the driving force that extends the legs.

Tip: Do not use momentum here. If you can't keep the motion controlled, decrease the weight.

Squats

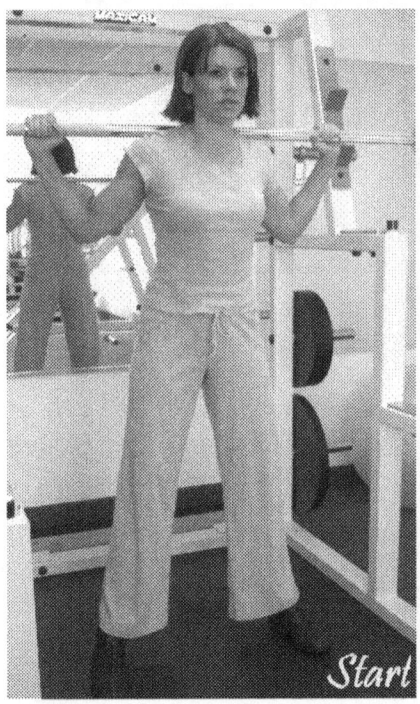
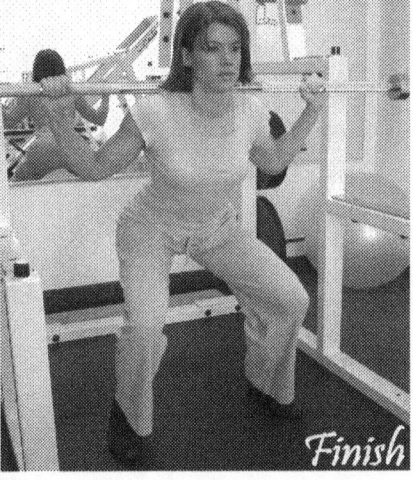

Center the bar on your upper back so that the weight is evenly distributed. Stand with your shoulders back, leaning forward slightly, knees slightly bent, and feet placed shoulder width apart. Slowly lower down, as if you were going to sit in a chair. Stop just before 90 degrees with the legs and push back up to starting position. Repeat.

Tip: If you can't come down very far, that's ok. Remember good form is everything. Also, make sure the weight is not too heavy.

Smith Machine Lunges

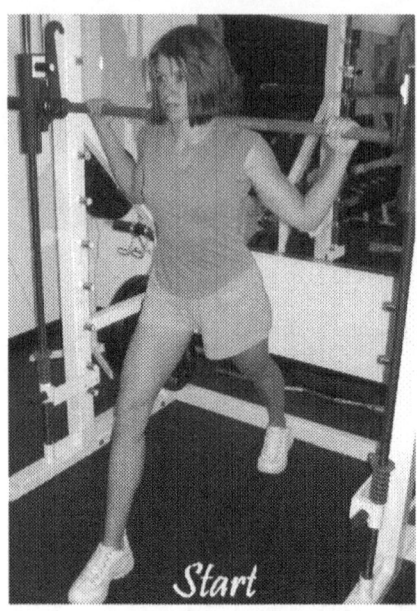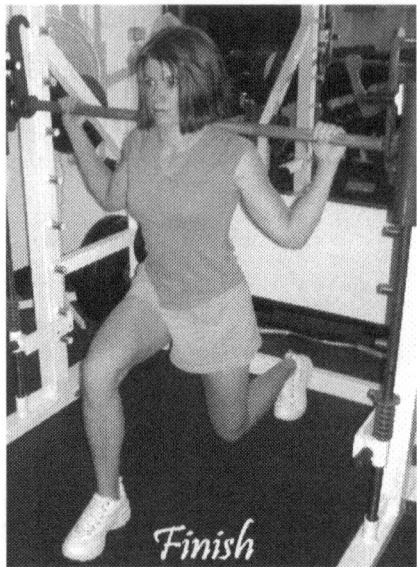

Stand centered under the bar on the Smith Machine. Lift the bar up and lock into place. Bring one leg forward, and step back with the opposite leg. Make sure that you have a wide stance for this exercise, so that the front knee doesn't go over the toe. Slowly lower the bar down, bending the back knee and lowering towards the floor. Push back up through the front leg to starting position. Repeat.

Tip: Keep the knees slightly bent at the top of the movement or starting position.

Hamstrings, Buns & Calves

Hamstring Curls

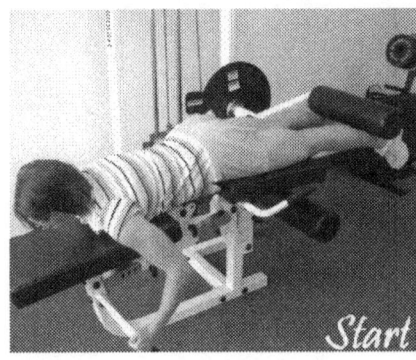
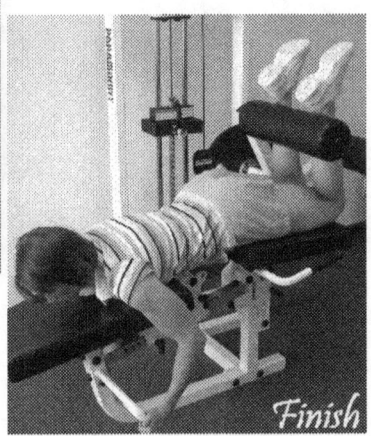

Lie face down on the leg curl machine so that your entire upper body and back is down. Place heels behind pad. Slowly curl the heels toward the buns so that you are contracting the back of the legs. Hold momentarily, and return to starting position but do not release weight. Repeat.

Tip: If you are really arching your back to try to get the weight up, then it's too heavy.

Reverse leg extensions

Use the leg attachment for the cable machine. Wrap around the ankle and secure firmly. Set the weight fairly low (5 to 10 pounds). Hold lightly on hand support rails for balance. Lean forward slightly and keep the supporting leg slightly bent at the knee. Slowly extend the working leg back, contracting the buns. Return to starting position, but do not release weight. Repeat.

Tip: This exercise is primarily for the buns, so make sure you are really contracting or squeezing the buns at the top of the movement.

Seated Calf Raises

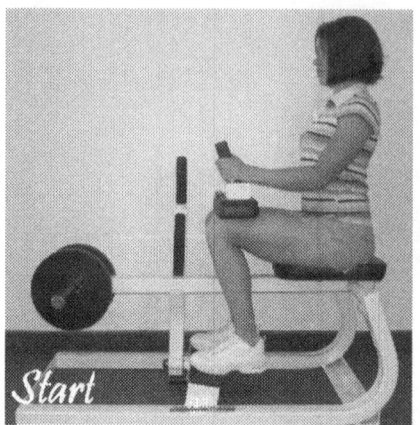 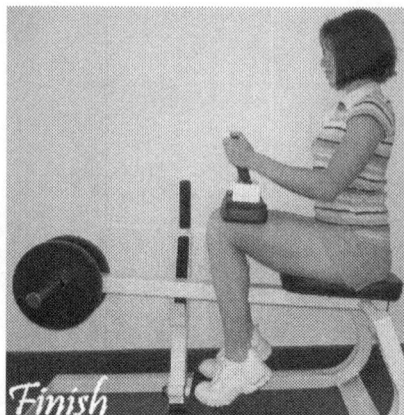

Place your knees firmly under the top pads for support and position the front of the feet on the bottom platform. Push up through the calf muscles and onto the top of the toes and contract the calf muscles. Slowly lower down so that the heels go slightly below the platform. Repeat movement.

Leg Press Calf Variation

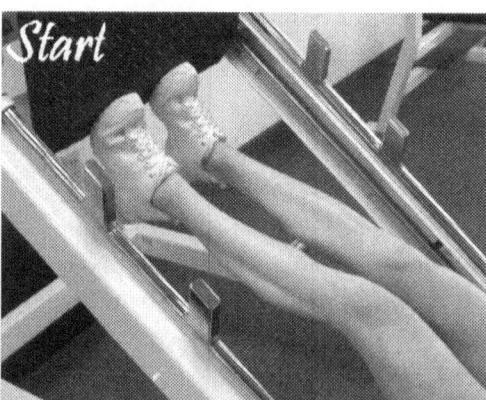

Place the front of the feet firmly against the bottom of the leg press platform, or use the calf platform if there is one. Keep the knees slightly bent and push the platform up and contract the calf muscles. Come back down to starting position, but don't use the legs, only the feet.

Tip: The knees stay slightly bent and stationary. The movement is only in the foot and ankle.

Shoulders

Smith Machine Shoulder Press

Use an incline bench and place in the full upright position. Position the bench so that the bar is fairly close to your face. Push bar up so that arms are fully extended overhead. Slowly lower down to shoulder level and repeat.

Tip: Keep hands in place during the movement so that the bar stays in unlocked position.

Smith Machine Upright Rows

Stand with feet shoulder width apart and knees slightly bent. Keep hands fairly close together and comfortably grip the bar. Raise the bar up to the chin, leading with the elbows. Slowly lower back down to starting position and repeat.

Tip: Make sure that the elbows are higher than the bar. Try not to use momentum, if you are arching your back excessively, lower the weight.

Variation: You may perform this exercise with the straight bar attachment at the cable machine.

Cable Front Raises

Using the rope attachment at lowest position, stand facing other side of machine, keep the shoulders back and knees slightly bent. Keeping the arms slightly bent, raise the arms up, separating the ends of the rope slightly. Raise arms up to shoulder level. Hold momentarily and return to starting position and repeat.

Tip: Don't lock the arms out at the elbows. Keep arms almost straight throughout the exercise.

Cable Side Raises

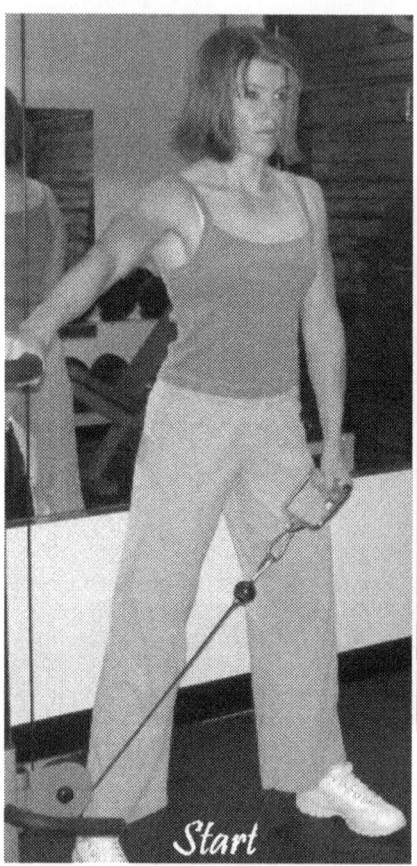
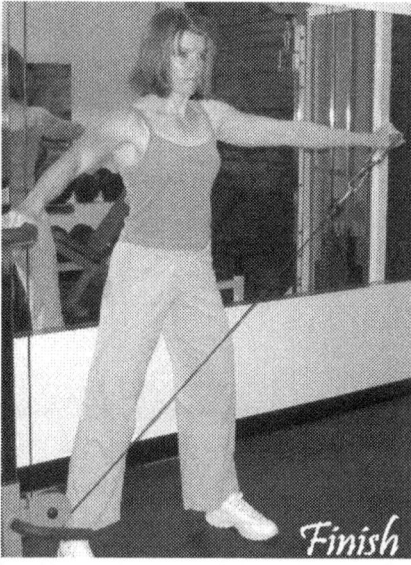

Using the single handle attachment at the lowest position, stand with feet apart and knees slightly bent. Slowly extend the working arm out to the side and up to shoulder level keeping the palm facing the floor. Slowly return to starting position and repeat.

Tip: Keep the elbow slightly bent and avoid using any momentum.

Chest

Bench Press

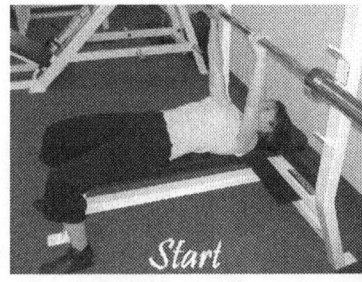 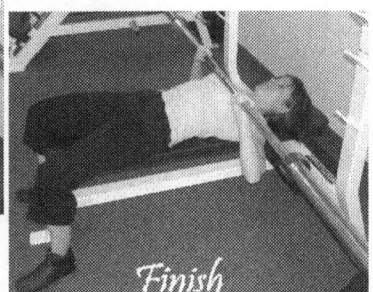

Lie flat on the bench and place hands shoulder width apart on the bar. Lift up to release bar from rack. Bending at the elbows, slowly lower down to the center of the chest and push back up through the chest. Repeat.

Tip: If possible, have someone spot you on this exercise.

Tip: If you feel yourself excessively arching your back, lower the weight.

Cable Crossovers

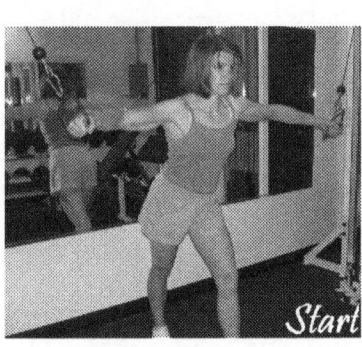 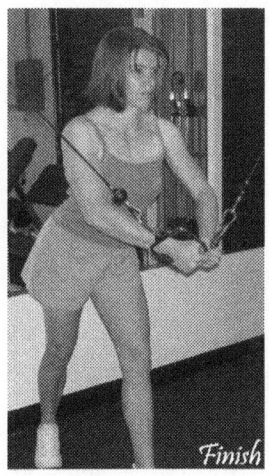

Use both handle attachments and adjust the cable to the highest position. Stand centered and position one foot forward and one slightly back. Lean forward slightly. Keeping the arms slightly bent, bring handles together in front of you and contract or squeeze the chest muscles. Slowly return to starting position and repeat.

Back

Pull Downs

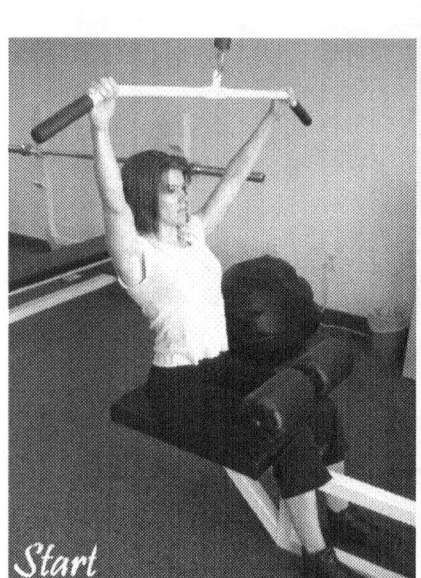
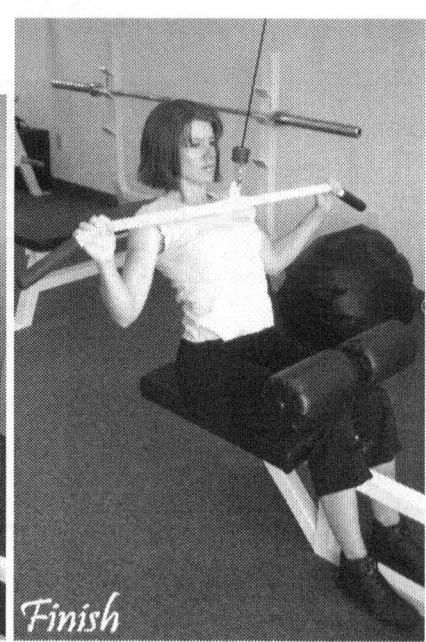

Place hands on the bar wider than shoulder width apart. Sit with knees firmly under pad. Push the chest up and out so that you have a slight arch in the back. Slowly pull the bar down towards the top of the chest, contracting the mid and upper back at the bottom of the movement. Slowly return to starting position and repeat.

Tip: Do not use any momentum here. This should be a smooth, controlled movement.

Tip: Think of bringing the elbows together at the bottom of the movement to contract the back muscles.

Seated Rows

At the seated row machine, reach forward to get the row attachment. Push the chest up and out so that you have a slight arch in the back. Keeping the arms close to the body, pull the attachment toward your midsection and contract or squeeze the mid back muscles. Slowly return to the starting position and repeat.

Tip: Keep the proper form at all times. Do not let the weight pull you forward.

One Arm Cable Rows

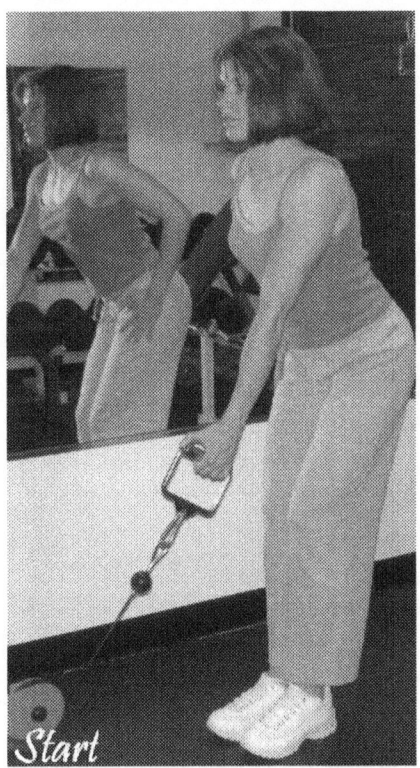 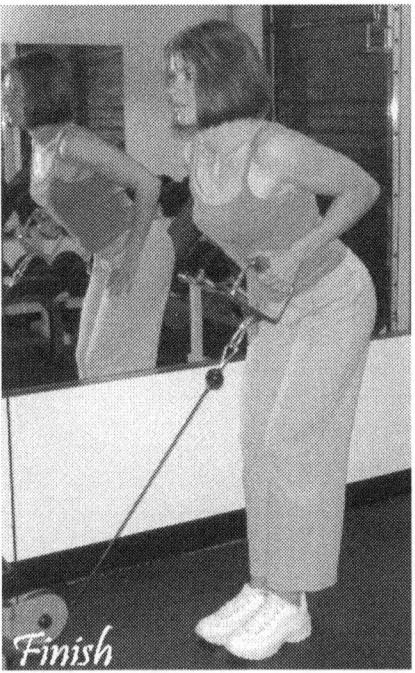

Use the single handle attachment and adjust cable to bottom position. Lean forward keeping the back flat and the chest up and out. Keeping the arm close to the body, slowly pull the handle back, contracting the mid back muscles. Return to starting position and repeat.

Tip: Make sure that you are leaning forward and your back is very flat.

Home Workout Rotation

Monday

Biceps	Triceps
Do 2 to 3 sets of 8 to 10 repetitions per set:	*Do 2 to 3 sets of 8 to 10 repetitions per set:*
• Barbell Curls • 21's - 2 to 3 sets, 21 repetitions each set. -or- • Dumbbell Curls • One Arm Isolation Curls (Incline bench)	• Lying Triceps extensions (Skull Crushers) • Dips • One Arm Extensions -or- • Triangle Pushups • Dips

Wednesday

Legs	Hamstrings
Do 2 to 3 sets with 10 to 15 reps per set.	*Do 2 to 3 sets with 10 to 15 reps per set.*
• Stationary Lunges • Reverse Lunges • Wall Squats -or- • Walking Lunges • Inner Thigh Squats • Alternating Lunges	• Dead Lifts • Standing Hamstring Curls -or- • Lying Hamstring Curls • Hamstring Squeeze **Calves** *Do 2 to 3 sets with 10 to 15 reps per set.* • Standing Calf Raise (on edge of stair)—Vary foot positions: Feet straight, toes inward, and toes outward.

Friday

Shoulders	Chest
Do 2 to 3 sets with 8 to 10 reps per set.	*Do 2 to 3 sets with 8 to 10 reps per set.*
• Military Press • Upright Rows-(dumbbells) • Side Raises • Seated Rear Shoulder Raises -or- • Pushups (shoulder width hand placement) • Upright Rows-(bar) • Front Raises • Side Raises	• Dumbbell Press (incline or flat bench) • Dumbbell Flys (incline or flat bench) -or- • Pushups • Dumbbell Flys (incline or flat bench) **Back** *Do 2 to 3 sets with 8 to 10 reps per set.* • One Arm Rows

Gym Workout Rotation

Monday

Biceps *Do 2 to 3 sets of 8 to 10 repetitions per set:*	Triceps *Do 2 to 3 sets of 8 to 10 repetitions per set:*
• Preacher Curls • 21's-(2 to 3 sets, 21 reps per set) • One Arm Cable Curls -or- • One Arm Isolation Curls • Standing Cable Curls • Barbell Curls	• Lying Triceps extensions (Skull Crushers) • One Arm Cable Extensions • Triangles -or- • Overhead Extensions-(cable) • Triceps Pushdowns • Dips

Wednesday

Legs *Do 2 to 3 sets with 10 to 15 reps per set.*	Hamstrings *Do 2 to 3 sets with 10 to 15 reps per set.*
• Smith Machine Lunges • Inner Thigh Squats • Squats -or- • Leg Extensions • Walking Lunges • Leg Press	• Hamstring Curls-(machine) • Hamstring Squeeze -or- • Dead Lifts • Standing Hamstring Curls **Calves** *Do 2 to 3 sets with 10 to 15 reps per set.* • Seated Calf Raise -or- • Leg Press Calf Variation

Friday

Shoulders	Chest
Do 2 to 3 sets with 8 to 10 reps per set.	*Do 2 to 3 sets with 8 to 10 reps per set.*
• Military Press-(Smith Machine) • Upright Rows-(Smith Machine) • Front Raises-(Cable/Rope) • Side Raises-(dumbbells) -or- • Seated Military Press-(dumbbells) • Upright Rows (dumbbells) • Cable or Dumbbell Side Raises • Seated Rear Shoulder Raises	• Bench Press • Dumbbell Flys (incline or flat bench) -or- • Dumbbell Press (incline or flat bench) • Cable Crossovers **Back** *Do 2 to 3 sets with 8 to 10 reps per set.* • One Arm Rows-(cable) • Pull downs -or- • Seated Rows • Pull downs

Benefits of Personal Training

Personal training has many advantages. Instruction, motivation, support, and accountability are the main reasons people seek out personal trainers. However, just because someone advertises themselves as a personal trainer doesn't mean that they have the qualifications necessary to ensure you proper, professional instruction. Do your research. Find out what certification(s) they have. While most states do not require any certification or licensure, it is to your benefit to find someone who is certified. The American Council on Exercise (ACE), International Sports Science Association (ISSA), and the American College of Sports Medicine (ACSM) are the most noteworthy.

Also, find out how long the trainer has been in business and how long they have been working out personally. This is a very important factor. Just as you wouldn't want a dentist that didn't take care of his own teeth, you wouldn't want a trainer who doesn't work out or look like they've ever touched a weight before. Find someone who practices what they preach!

Price range varies considerably, but the average is around $50 per hour. Don't necessarily opt for the trainer who charges more, unless their qualifications and background are directly related to the price. And don't look for the cheap way out. Remember, you get what you pay for.

If you feel that you would be well suited working with a personal trainer, spend some time interviewing until you feel that you have a good match. A good trainer should be willing to allow you an initial consultation, free of charge, and answer any questions that you have about weight loss and fitness. He or she should be courteous, prompt, motivating, and understanding. The trainer should be knowledgeable, but if he or she can't answer your question(s), then be willing to refer you in the right direction instead of guessing or making something up.

The trainer should also do a fairly comprehensive health screening to determine if you are a good candidate. If you feel someone is too pushy or lacks interest, go somewhere else. After all, it's *your* investment! A good trainer will make sure that it is money well spent.

Work Out Like a Pro

We've all seen the magazine ads or television shows with models that look like they were sculpted from stone. So, what's the *real* secret to building a sculpted body? Great genetics? Nope. You guessed it, ***consistency***! Don't take my word for it. Ask anyone who works out with weights. Professional bodybuilders and fitness models will tell you that good workouts and proper nutrition are the cornerstones for weight loss and fitness success. It doesn't happen overnight, but the results are worth every bit of work.

So now you have the basics of nutrition and resistance training, and you're ready to embark on your transformation. I want you to make each and every workout session worthwhile. Here are some helpful tips to keep you progressing at a steady pace.

1. Always schedule your workouts in your day and make them priority!

Just as you wouldn't miss a doctor's appointment or your hairdresser's appointment, neither should you miss your workout appointment. Even if you aren't going to be using a trainer, schedule your workouts and be there ready to go on time!

2. Keep track of your daily workout routines.

Don't spend too much time on this, remember, you want to keep your rest times minimal. Just make a chart that allows you to quickly note the exercise, amount of weight, number of sets, and approximate repetitions per set. Do this for the first 2 to 4 weeks, depending on your comfort level. After that, you should be able to do your routine without keeping record. This will greatly increase your overall workout productivity.

3. Following your warm up set, do your heaviest set first. Challenge yourself! Heavier weights mean better, faster results.

I want you to focus on heavier weights with proper form. A good way to determine if you are using heavy enough weights is to do 10 repetitions. If you can do 10 easily, then your weights are too light. If you are finding it challenging, but keeping good form and really pushing to get 10 reps, you are in the right area. Your next set should be a little less intense and you should be getting around 10 to 12 repetitions per set.

4. Find a workout partner.

A good workout partner can make a big difference in your performance. He or she can assist or spot you on the heavy sets, and help you stay motivated on the days that you don't feel like doing anything. However, make sure that you find someone who is likeminded and serious about the workout. If you have someone who would rather talk than work out, you're better off by yourself. If you aren't interested in having a partner, that's okay too. Make sure you are pushing yourself and staying challenged.

5. Stay informed.

This book will give you a great start to your fitness routine. All of the exercises given can be adjusted to be more challenging as your strength and endurance progresses. It is to your benefit to learn, whether in magazines or books, additional new exercises to add to your routine. Variety is key. Experiment with different exercises and change your routines regularly. Remember, you want to keep the body guessing.

6. Do measurements.

It is extremely important to track your progress for motivation and accountability. This can be done various ways, such as body fat measurements, clothing, tape measurements, and pictures. It is highly recommended that you do all of these to see the most change. Keep this information in your journal along with your before and after photos. I recommend doing a *progress check up* every 4 to 6 weeks. If you don't have a personal trainer, body composition tests such as body fat assessment, can be done at your local health club.

7. Stay focused and continue to visualize.

I discussed earlier the importance of visualization. Never stop visualizing. If you have met your goals or are approaching them, reevaluate. Find new, more challenging goals to set your sights on. This mental focus is absolutely imperative to your continued success.

Chapter 7

Adjusting the Plan to Your Progress

Changing Your Food Intake to Accommodate Your Weight Loss

When you approach your particular weight loss goal, you can now incorporate various foods into your plan to help maintain your results. Here are some basic guidelines to follow to adjust the plan to your needs.

You may:

1. Gradually increase protein portion size. In this case you can add 2 to 3 ounces of extra protein at each meal. This increase in protein intake will be necessary as you continue to build your muscle mass.

2. Moderate certain foods. Below is a list of suggested foods that you can add into the plan. **Limit these foods to one serving, 3 to 4 times per week.**

<u>Food</u>	<u>Serving Size</u>
Applesauce	½ cup
Beans	½ cup
Whole grain bread	1 additional slice
Corn on the cob	½ medium cob
Corn tortilla	2 small tortillas
Whole egg	1 additional egg
Fruit	½ cup or small to medium serving of fresh fruit
Dried fruit	½ cup
Assorted nuts	¼ cup
Pastas	½ cup cooked serving
Peanut butter	1 tablespoon low fat variety
Pretzels	½ cup
White rice or other varieties	½ cup cooked

The main emphasis is to gradually increase the overall caloric intake and increase the variety in your plan. If you find that you'd rather stick to the regular plan and save the other foods for your day off, then increase portion sizes at each meal by ¼ more of everything. Continue to eat every 3 hours, and make sure water intake stays at 1 gallon per day.

The body requires more calories for energy as you increase your overall lean muscle mass. As your body fat continues to decrease because of the shift from fat to muscle, you will need to increase your caloric intake. If you don't increase your calories from food, your body will resort to slowly depleting your hard-earned muscle mass. Gradually adjust your portion sizes and incorporate some new foods into your daily intake and your body will adjust accordingly.

For those of you that have minimal to no desired body fat weight to lose, this plan will work for you also. The goal, whether you are trying to lose weight or not, is to increase your overall lean muscle mass. In doing so, you will still need to eat clean and frequently. However, portion size should increase by ¼ more of everything. Also, dietary fat and carbohydrate intake are not as strict in this circumstance. You should include foods from the above list everyday to the regular plan. You should also take the recommended day off.

Challenging Yourself in Your Workouts

Just as it's necessary to modify your dietary intake as you progress, but also in your workouts. It is very easy to *plateau* in your workout routines. While you may find it easy to maintain your body composition doing the same exercises and amount of weight that you find comfortable, you will not continue to see dramatic results. It is necessary to increase your *intensity* whenever possible. This might mean getting a couple extra repetitions that you wouldn't normally be able to do or taking a decreased rest time. Little things like that are what are required to keep moving forward.

Visualization increases intensity. I want you to take visualization a step further during your workouts. Start to visualize the muscle working and contracting. Think about the exercise and eliminate all momentum. Each movement should be smooth and controlled. Every motion, both positive and negative, has a unique purpose. Incorporate this attention to detail into your workouts and I promise you will eliminate any plateau.

Make sure that you are keeping your workout routines fresh. I have included a rotation of exercises in both workout plans that you should alternate every week. Make sure that you aren't going through the motions during your sessions. Mix things up by changing your music regularly and possibly working out with a partner 2 to 3 times per week. Most importantly, make your workouts fun and stimulating!

Overcoming Plateaus

As you continue to progress with the plan, you may occasionally feel as if your body fat loss is slowing down or at a plateau. Do not be discouraged! This is a last ditch effort for your body to try to spare its body fat and it is quite normal. Make sure you are keeping your workouts intense and you are religiously eating clean and frequently. This is just a temporary phase. The continual increase in lean muscle mass will increase your metabolic rate an offset any plateau. Continue to follow the plan and keep your head high—consistency will always prevail!

Chapter 8

Why You Will See Better Results—*Year After Year!*

Increasing Your Calorie Burning Efficiency

The beautiful thing about staying consistent with your workouts and eating is that your results will get better and better. Basically, your body will continue to refine and increase its lean muscle mass. You will notice definition and shape becoming more prominent. Your body is continually adapting to the work you are challenging it to do.

As you continue to increase your muscle mass, even as gradual as it may be, you are also increasing your overall resting metabolic rate and calorie burning efficiency. The metabolism will continue to do this as long as you stay consistent. You will find that you will have more flexibility with eating higher calorie foods through the week. The increase in caloric demands from your body will welcome this change in eating. Be certain, however, that you moderate your intake of higher caloric foods and still save the pizza and ice cream for your day off!

Muscle Maturity

The process of refining the muscle mass and increasing shape, size, and definition over time is referred to as *muscle maturity*. For the most part, everyone has a different baseline or starting point when in the beginning stages of muscle growth. There are several factors that determine the size and shape of your muscles such as genetics, age, and activity level. However, no matter what your genetic predisposition or age, you can still build good, quality lean muscle mass. It is the consistency of good quality workouts and proper nutrition over time that makes the real changes in muscle development.

As I mentioned before, a 60-year-old woman that has been weight training consistently for 10 years will look dramatically different than a 30-year-old woman who has been sedentary and is just starting a weight training program. It is important to note here that proper nutrition over time also plays a key role in muscle growth and maturity.

A Lifestyle You Can Live With and Love!

If you've learned anything about this program, I hope it's that *diets just don't work*. The changes you want to make have to come from within yourself, and it has to be something you can truly live with. It's time to stop depriving and punishing yourself with food. Start learning how to really care for your body, mind, and spirit.

Starting the program is just the beginning. This should be a lifelong commitment to better health and fitness. If it isn't, you won't succeed, and that's the truth. The key to staying motivated and on track is to find that balance. This program combines just that, balanced nutrition and balanced workouts.

You will find as you go along, eating properly will become easier and routine. Your body will begin to stop craving unhealthy foods, as long as you are consistently eating clean. You will find your day off will probably become less and less about eating everything and anything you want, just because you can, but rather about eating something you *enjoy*. Your workouts should become more intense, and you will find your recovery times decreasing. Your noticeable results will ignite a deeper passion to keep pushing yourself. You will create a much healthier, happier life, and become a role model for others. Take charge today and start this program tomorrow, you will not regret it!

Setting New Goals

I have discussed the importance of goals in your life. Make sure you *always* have goals. As soon as you meet your goals, make sure you set new ones, both short and long term. Don't underestimate the power of setting goals. The sky is the limit. No matter how small or large, practical or unrealistic, always have them. You will be amazed at how easy it really is to meet them. But you will never know, until you try.

Ok, that's that. My question to you is—what are *you* waiting for?

> *"The future belongs to those who believe in the beauty of their dreams."*
> —*Eleanor Roosevelt*

To learn more about Lauren's program, please visit www.donewithdieting.com

About the Author

Lauren Shaw is certified by the American Council on Exercise (ACE) as a Personal Trainer, Lifestyle & Weight Management Consultant, and Group Fitness Instructor. She has a background in physical rehabilitation therapy as well as Biology. She has avidly been involved in the health and fitness industry for over ten years. Her philosophy is based on all natural nutrition and resistance training.

Lauren and her fiancé, Rick, own and operate Physique Transformations Studio, a personal training studio in Colorado Springs, Colorado. She enjoys spending time with Rick and her dog Taylor, and also enjoys hiking, power walking, and camping.

0-595-33525-X